Advance Pr<del>a</del>

In Thriving through Cancer, Kelly writes with deep understanding of what many experience in cancer care: a vacuum in supportive nutrition and lifestyle recommendations. Through the functional medicine lens, this book inspires incorporation of whole-istic pillars to cancer care with soothing guidance, introspection, and unique application to oneself. Cancer diagnosis and treatment can create many uncertainties; however, the author empowers readers with reliable, foundational choices to help create a profoundly different cancer care experience: one of thriving versus surviving. As an oncology RN, I highly recommend choosing this book as a 'teammate' in your cancer care.

— **Zenia Irani**, MSN, RN

Thriving Through Cancer by Kelly Lutman is an essential resource for those seeking a holistic approach to cancer management. This insightful and informative book presents practical dietary advice with an emphasis on the healing aspects of nutrition. An inspiring and empowering read for anyone looking to achieve optimal wellness during and after a cancer diagnosis.

— **Eleanore Goldstein**, RN

This book understands a cancer diagnosis as it should be. A thoughtful, understanding functional medicine coaching perspective that focuses on more than just one approach to treatment and education. Kelly does a tremendous job at providing hope through using rational explanations for a better quality of life and not just more statistics. *Thriving Through Cancer* is a must read for anyone affected by cancer. If you or your loved ones have been looking deeper into understanding cancer, read this book.

— **Michael Reid**, functional oncology coach and founder, HealthAsMeant2B

When you are faced with the reality that you have cancer, there is a firehose of information coming your way but information about how nutrition will help you is lacking. Kelly's book provides a balance of relevant stories, science, and guidance to express her insight. It's this approach that helps you understand why nutrition matters so much at this critical time. I also appreciate that she reinforces that the choice of what you integrate is up to you. This no-pressure, informative guide is a must-read for those walking through their own cancer journey.

—**J.M. Frustaci**, cancer Survivor

Thriving Through Cancer: A Whole-istic Approach for Your Journey by Kelly Lutman is a book that provides a comprehensive approach to cancer treatment. What I find particularly captivating is Kelly's perspective on how the book can become your "guide on this nourishing journey" —powerful word choices that highlight the importance of nourishing the body during cancer treatment, rather than just following a restrictive cancer diet.

Kelly explains how the body already has an intricate approach to fighting diseases, including cancer, but it needs the right nutrients to function optimally.

In summary, this book is a must-read for cancer patients, their loved ones, and anyone interested in taking a holistic approach to cancer treatment. It offers a wealth of valuable insights and practical guidance that can make a real difference in one's cancer journey.

— **Ewa Andrykiewicz Zmyslona**, bestselling
author of *The Healing Mindset: How Cancer
Activated My 8 Superpowers*

If you or someone you know is dealing with a cancer diagnosis, I highly recommend reading *Thriving Through Cancer*. Using a wonderfully engaging narrative style for an emotionally difficult topic, Kelly provides valuable insight on adding a holistic approach to treating cancer. She offers strategies for nutritional support as well as for improving physical, emotional, and spiritual well-being to nourish the body. With engaging writing and great use of analogies, this book is sure to empower and inspire those dealing with or supporting someone with a cancer diagnosis, offering an informative and uplifting approach to the journey of recovery.

— **Sybil Cooper**, Ph.D.

In *Thriving Through Cancer*, the language and writing style are extremely clear and easy to follow, without being patronizing—especially for a non-native English speaker. It is obvious that Kelly Lutman has a huge knowledge in her field and also a sincere wish to help her audience. She is on a mission. While many books on illnesses are focused on treating the illness, Kelly's focus is on healing the people, and there is much love between the lines.

— **Hanne Brøter**, author of *Brand Boxes*

Thriving through Cancer provides encouragement and empowerment to those in the trenches of their cancer journey. This book offers a holistic blueprint for true healing, addressing the body's physical and nutritional needs as well as the health of the mind and spirit. Kelly Lutman clearly communicates information and expert guidance to enable those diagnosed with cancer as well as their caregivers to say farewell to a state of survival and enter a life of thriving through their circumstances.

— **Megan Roberts**, FNP-C

Several people I love have had to navigate a cancer diagnosis. While each of their experiences has been unique, they have all suffered from the side effects of treatment needed to save their lives. When I heard about this book, I knew I wanted to share it with them right away! Here are powerful actions they can implement on their own to help them both feel better and regain a sense of control. This book addresses the whole patient —mind, body, and spirit—and infuses a challenging journey with the beauty of hope.

— **Stacy Rowan**, human design & mindset coach

A must-have resource for anyone who has received a cancer diagnosis. Just the right amount of science, in simple terms, to explain the facts behind the recommendations. A primer for taking control of things you can control—what you eat and think—when going through a treatment plan for cancer. Scant nutrition advice is offered by doctors and what is offered does little to bolster the body against the attack on the body during cancer treatment. A must-read for yourself, family, friends, or anyone wanting to take control and face cancer head on.

— **Connie Jo Miller**, author of
Words of Whimsy trilogy

An enlightening look at the benefits of an integrative and holistic approach for cancer patients to align body, mind and soul to heal. Drawing upon her experience as a certified health coach and functional medicine practitioner, Kelly Lutman offers her expertise as a nutrition expert to provide easy to implement steps that support the body's immune system to complement and enhance traditional cancer treatments.

— **Leslie Lawrence**, author of
*I'm a Lucky Woman! A Photographic Memoir of a
Breast Cancer Survivor*

I wish this kind of help had been available when my mother was being treated for cancer! Kelly Lutman brings home the value of proper nutrition during cancer treatment to getting through the treatment phase and aiding in a faster recovery. And the advice is fantastic even if you don't have a cancer diagnosis! Finding the right foods for your own optimal health is an adventure worth undertaking.

— **Cheri D. Andrews, Esq.**, author of
*Smooth Sailing: A Practical Guide to
Legally Protecting Your Business*

Thriving Through Cancer is the book I wish I had for my mother, who passed away from breast cancer in 2022. Mom was incredibly concerned about her nutrition during her cancer treatment, and she told me several times that she wished she had better nutritional resources to refer to. Kelly Lutman's book is the answer that so many cancer patients need!

—**Jill Celeste, MA**, author of
Loud Woman: Good-bye, Inner Good Girl!

As a board-certified colon hydrotherapist, I understand how important nutrition and digestion are to the overall function of the body. Kelly takes it one step further and easily explains how this is different for every single person. Understanding the need to nourish the body's cells for health is key to each person's journey to health and wellness, whether thriving through cancer or living life to the fullest. I love the way Kelly explains this in terms that are not judgmental or off-putting, and I look forward to the book being released so I can read the rest of it and share it with my clients. Thanks for sharing your journey and knowledge, Kelly. It's amazing!

— **Cathy Agasar**, I-ACT certified colon
hydrotherapist and bestselling author of
The Gift of Loss

An affirming, supportive, and educational resource for anyone on a journey with cancer. Kelly has knowledge and compassion in spades, and a passion for keeping you in the driver's seat of your experience.

— **Vanden-Pilar Moseley**, board-
certified health coach

This book provides a wealth of information about the body, its digestion needs and processes, and how to create support for a body that is combatting cancer. Coming from a functional nutrition perspective, and including mindset, movement, and sleep advice as well, the author covers a broad range of topics designed to help people win that war.

—**Judy Kane**, founder, Aligned Consciousness,
and author of *Your4Truths:
How Beliefs Impact Your Life*

Mrs. Lutman shares her tremendous knowledge about the importance of nutrition and the healing it bestows on our bodies. She makes an excellent case for the often-overlooked value of nutrition in the fight against cancer. She writes as though she is speaking to a friend. Her words are very calming and gives the reader real hope. This book will be of benefit to everyone that reads it.

— **Elizabeth Nelson**, author of
In the Shadow of Your Wings, A Journey

I believe this book will be an incredible resource for anyone diagnosed with cancer as a step-by-step guide on the journey to thrive through an extremely taxing illness and attack on the human body. The most encouraging part of this book is that it teaches people that they can thrive during the journey instead of merely surviving it. As a practicing registered dental hygienist, I've had several patients describe the same dilemma after being diagnosed with cancer and given very little if any nutritional information or education. This book provides an excellent guide and act as a health compass for all those on this difficult road to be able to THRIVE.

— **Tiffany Magee**, registered dental hygienist

This book is eye-opening about the role of food and nutrition in health, and in particular for thriving through cancer. It's a must-read for anyone recently diagnosed with cancer and their family and friends. And I'd say it's a must-read for anyone involved with treating cancer too—oncologists, nurses, and other health professionals need to understand more about how nutrition can affect their patients. I wish this book had been around when my Dad was going through his treatments for stomach cancer.

— **Catherine Williams**, CEO,
Chapter One Book Production

In *Thriving Through Cancer*, Kelly Lutman clearly and compassionately outlines how everyone fighting cancer—and their loved ones—can flip the script on cancer to reduce the side effects and speed your healing. Her practical, holistic, whole person advice is the missing piece that complements medical cancer treatment and increases your resilience.

— **Mary Foley**, podcast host of
Live Like Your Nail Color

Brava to Kelly Lutman for providing guidance and high-lighting healthy options for anyone impacted by cancer. Her expertise in the field of wellness shines brightly in this amazing guide that truly speaks to the positive impact food has on health.

— **Gina Ramsey**, author of *Burnt Gloveboxes*

One's struggle with cancer requires all aspects of the individual's body to be involved. I love the way Kelly has brought mind, body and soul together to defeat cancer. I really wish that I had had this book for my own cancer journey.

— **Wanda Padgett**, cancer survivor

Thriving Through Cancer

believing in your
body's resilience!
Kelly Litman

Thriving Through Cancer
A Whole-istic Approach for Your Journey

Kelly Lutman, AFMC

Edited by
Deborah Kevin

HIGHLANDER
PRESS

ISBN: 978-1-956442-17-5
Ebook ISBN: 978-1-956442-18-2
Library of Congress Control Number: 2023938242

Published by Highlander Press
501 W. University Pkwy, Ste. B2
Baltimore, MD 21210

Cover design: Hanne Broter
Managing Editor: Deborah Kevin, MA
Author photo credit: Still Reflections Photography

Contents

To my beloved, Tom,
Thank you for believing in me and
encouraging me to follow my passion.

To my clients,
Who have proven how the body can heal when its building blocks are
maximized, what works against it is minimized, and a healing
environment is prioritized.

Introduction

Scanning the list of emails in my inbox, my eyes caught the name of a friend I hadn't heard from in a while. I knew she had been in treatment for breast cancer for a few months and I was eager to see whether this email would share how she was doing.

I was surprised by what I read:

> I knew that when the nutrition section of my two-inch binder for 'The Care and Feeding of the Cancer Patient' [a resource from her oncologist] included drinking Ensure and Carnation Instant Breakfast stuff, I was not being supported nutritionally. I want to invite in excellent supportive nutrition to counterbalance the medical interventions as much as humanly possible! I'm so glad you have expertise in this area!

I had heard stories of poor nutritional support for cancer patients but was surprised to hear the details of how bad it was. Yet, I was also encouraged that my friend had remembered what she had heard me share in the past and wanted my support on her care team.

Yes, I would help her! As a certified health coach and functional medicine practitioner, I would definitely be able to support her efforts to counterbalance the medical interventions so that her body could do more than survive. I wanted my friend to thrive!

My heart sank at the thought that my friend and other cancer patients—people in the battle for their life—were being told to drink products that really don't qualify as nourishment for their cells. In fact, these products could actually work against them in their battle. Inside me I felt the spark of a calling to not only help my friend but many others—including you—through the battle.

We may think of battles primarily in terms of soldiers on the front line, but there is so much more involved. Those soldiers need support in a wide range of areas as a foundation for their efforts. They need communication to enable them to find out what is happening around them and pass on information that they collect. They need transportation to and from the front line. They need supplies to continue their efforts and coordination with nearby units. And they need a plan to direct their efforts.

The same could be said for the body and its internal battle against disease. The frontline soldiers are white blood cells, part of your immune system, and they need the support of communication from your nerves and neurotransmitters. Your lymph system delivers these important immune cells to the battlefield and then helps clear debris. How well are the command controls working to support them and the units around them—the primary organs, the adrenal system, the circulatory system and more?

The body already has an intricately programmed approach for fighting disease, including the daily threats of microbes and chemicals that invade the body through food, air, water, and skin. When the body is supplied with what it needs to function optimally, it can handle both the intervention with daily threats and the resolution of disease. The key is to ensure the supply of nutrients is available.

When embarking on a journey into unfamiliar territory, it helps to have a guide or better yet, a team. You already have several medical guides and family members on your team. I would like to join your team as a nutrition expert, guiding your body's nourishment and supporting its battle against cancer. I can bridge a gap between the focus on the battle against cancer and the need to support the rest of your body as the battlefield.

I have supported many through the process of reclaiming their health after a wide variety of diagnoses. I use functional medicine principles to look at the body as a whole system and symptoms as messages the body is sending to indicate what isn't working properly. It is a science-based, root-cause focus on restoring function.

My own journey into health and functional medicine started with the realization that my son, whom I was homeschooling, had ADHD. I wasn't comfortable with simply getting a formal diagnosis and medication, so I began to search for information and found the work of Dr. Benjamin Feingold, a pediatric allergist. Dr. Feingold's theory was that hyperactivity was caused by allergic reaction to salicylates and artificial colors and flavors in food. Our family committed to his two-week protocol and were amazed to see significant change in my son's behavior. He was now able to sit and focus on his work, carry on a conversation with eye contact, and not seem driven to move constantly. And all we did was change our food.

That was my aha moment. It lit a spark in me that I fanned with further research about the powerful effect of food on the body. As the flame grew brighter, I pursued training in health coaching and functional medicine and embarked on a fresh mission to support others in pursuing wellness. I have worked with clients for nearly ten years and each of them has come to me with different circumstances. They may have had similar diagnoses—the names given to a collection of symptoms—but their unique bodies needed different interventions.

I will never forget my first client with cancer. Her name is Annie, and we got started after she had had surgery to remove a brain tumor but before she began radiation and chemotherapy. As we worked together—adjusting the foods she ate, and the ways she supported her body and her faith—she was able to go through the radiation treatments with very few symptoms. Her oncologist was so surprised at her lack of symptoms that he wanted to prescribe an antidepressant, assuming she was in denial. It wasn't denial. Annie was living a nourished life with hope.

Your body's systems work like an orchestra and when disease is at play, there are usually instruments (organs) that are out of tune or need cleaning. Though many would recognize the instruments, each are slightly unique, just as you as a whole are unique as well.

The sound of an orchestra varies with the balance of instruments and the musicians playing them, as well as the environment where it is playing. If in a concert hall, where acoustics have been engineered into the design, there will be a different sound than outdoors or in a small facility. Pursuing wellness is a bit like tuning instruments and adjusting the environment. It's not a quick fix, but the resulting balance is invigorating.

Naturally, we need to walk through the type of foods that will provide the nutrients your body needs for proper function, along with what modifications to make given the side effects of your treatment. But we won't stop there.

Your body is also heavily influenced by your thoughts, what you hear on a daily basis from both inside and outside, as well as your life experiences. Wellness is multidimensional, involving the integration of body, mind and spirit. True healing, therefore, requires addressing not only the body's need for nutrient supply, but also aspects of mind and spirit to find the roadblocks or detours that are contributing to disease. To this end, we will explore the mind-body connection, purpose, movement, and spirituality.

You didn't pick up this book by accident. Even if it was a gift from a friend or family member, you made the choice to open it and skim through the beginning pages. That tells me you are looking for a better way, a way to provide the "excellent supportive nutrition" for your whole body that my friend referenced in her message.

Having interviewed many who are currently or have recently been in cancer treatment, I recognize that side effects from treatment may influence whether you are comfortable with reading. I will be providing video resources and handouts, as well as keep the chapters short so that you have multiple ways to learn how to support your body.

I firmly believe in the body's ability to overcome obstacles—to heal—when given the building blocks that it needs for optimal function. I want you to be equipped to THRIVE rather than simply survive. It is my sincere hope that in reading this book, you will find portions that you can integrate for your life. Let's be honest, you won't experience a different outcome if you don't make changes. Yet, once you make those changes consistently, I know that you will begin to see that your body is amazing, and that healing—indeed, wellness —is entirely possible.

As Water Flows

Have you ever found yourself sitting by a body of water —whether a stream or river or even the ocean—watching the manner in which water flows? It fills space, creeping around objects that resist it and seeking a way into new territory. Water takes the shape of whatever container it occupies, be it natural or manmade.

It can change its form between rigid ice, nebulous steam or fluid liquid, yet it never changes its true nature. Water is both resilient and persistent. Given time, it carves or drips its mark into its environment. The Grand Canyon and mighty stalactites found in caves are clear evidence of water's impression and the beauty it leaves behind.

Some of us learned to be like water early in life while others are still fighting the direction our life's current is taking us. Amy Montemarano, writer and world traveler, has learned in living with Parkinson's disease that "being like water means having the ability to flow in whatever direction and into whatever container our life situation hands us. It doesn't change our lives' difficulties, but it allows us to stop struggling and deal with any situation from an authentic place."

She continues, "If we constantly fight our life situation and try to force it into the shape we want, we get frustrated, angry, anxious, and scared." We push against obstacles that we can't influence. What we can influence is our perspective.

As you explore your options in this journey, you get to choose your path and your perspective. Many will offer their recommendations, some may even be rather forceful in their opinion, yet the choice is still yours. If a fast and aggressive approach resonates with you, hit it. And if you feel the need to take more time to pursue the end goal, seek support in doing that. The same goes with the recommendations shared in this book. They represent many ways to support your body, mind and spirit, yet the choice of what you will integrate in your journey is yours.

Will you be reactive or proactive along the way? There will certainly be occasions where an unexpected turn of events will require a reactive decision but focusing on a proactive approach in supporting the whole of your being will give you firmer footing.

My sons played basketball in their high school years. Unlike in many sports where there are specifically offensive and defensive players, those who play basketball must switch back and forth. When they are in possession of the ball, they work together to move the ball down the court toward the goal. One player rarely takes it all the way alone. A more effective approach is to pass the ball back and forth to work around the other team's players.

One unexpected move can shift the play in the other direction and those players who were moving toward their own goal, now have to defend against the other team's effort to score. There's an amazing fluidity to the game, moving like water around obstacles in a stream. And occasionally you will see a team call time out and they will confer on the sidelines to determine an alternate approach.

You will no doubt experience both the shift between offense and defense—being proactive or reactive—but you have the benefit of maintaining possession of the ball.

Who is on the bench for your team? You may have some team members who were selected for you, and others that you can recruit.

It is important that you feel your team members are on your side and you communicate well. The additional recruits may be friends, family or practitioners that would help you counter the negative effects of traditional cancer treatment—I hope that you would count this book and its contents in that category.

You may read about methods of support in this book and be able to integrate them in your plan on your own, much like a basketball player uses fundamentals or special plays to improve performance. Or you may feel that you need a coach by your side to help you choose the plays and skills that will improve your game. Again, it's your choice.

Put into Action

What thoughts have come up as you read this chapter? Have you been playing offense or defense in your journey thus far? I encourage you to take a minute and write down your thoughts in response to what you have read and then write what you would like your journey to look like. Some would call this practice "setting an intention." When walking to a destination in the distance, you will arrive more directly if you fix your eyes on the destination rather than keeping them focused on the ground. Setting an intention, especially in writing, is like fixing your eyes on the destination. Yes, you will need to navigate things in front of you, but keep returning your focus on the desired destination.

Your Guide on
This Nourishment Journey

IF YOU WERE TO INTERVIEW ME AS YOUR NUTRITION GUIDE, what questions would you want to ask? Perhaps you would want to know more about the outcomes that my clients have experienced. Or you would want to know more about my training. Maybe your first question is if I will make you give up a food you love. Relax, I'm not your boss. You will retain the power of choice. I will simply educate you on the benefits or risks of some choices.

Let me first say that I didn't choose the path I am on. It seems to have chosen me. My original choice of profession was accounting, which I discovered an affinity for in high school. I was engaged to be married and wanted a profession with flexibility in case we had children. As it ends up, I decided to set accounting aside and homeschool my sons after teaching the middle one to read at four years old. I realized he would not be challenged appropriately if he went into a normal kindergarten classroom.

I've already shared about my son's ADHD—yes, it was the same son that also started our homeschool journey (he seems to have been instrumental in the directional changes of my life). Recognizing the power that food held over his body and behaviors was a tremendous eye-opener for me. Until that point, I had experienced the pleasures of food—primarily in taste and smell and texture—and knew that it was common to get sleepy after a big holiday meal. Yet, I did not recognize that food is also *information* for the body.

I also did not realize how truly unique each body is. Indeed, one man's food can be another man's poison, depending on how each body responds to the information provided. The concept of bio-individuality was driven home in my health coach training, and I studied a variety of dietary plans as tools in my toolbox to support individual people's needs. One diet does not fit every body, as evidenced by the wide range of dietary plans promoted on the market. I work with each of my clients to find the foods that nourish them in their unique body, and that sometimes shifts along their healing journey.

I worked with clients as a health coach for three years before starting my functional medicine training. While in school I continued to work with clients and incorporated what I was learning for their benefit. Clients began to come to me (and still do) with a range of more complex challenges and diagnoses. We adjusted the foods they were eating and the way they supported their bodies with movement and sleep. We explored how their relationships and careers were influencing their wellness, and how much joy they experienced in their lives. You see, it all works together! Step by step we peel the onion to find out what is working against them and provide what the body needs to function properly, and Type 2 Diabetes, Irritable Bowel Syndrome (IBS), Hashimoto's, achy joints and more are resolved.

Training in applied functional medicine opened my eyes to the amazing intricacies of the human body. My experience with conventional medicine had led me to see the body as a series of systems—cardiovascular, endocrine, skeletal, muscular, and more—which seemed somehow segregated. In reality, all of these systems are closely intertwined, with seemingly unrelated parts effecting others. Hit your thumb with a hammer and you will feel the effect in more

than your thumb! Suffer a concussion and, surprisingly, your digestion will also be hampered.

Functional medicine views the symptoms of the body as signals—
something like semaphore signals—the body uses to communicate its
need for support. My training helped me to learn to read those signals
and follow them upstream to the root of the problem. It could be
insufficient stomach acid that hinders the body's ability to break
protein down into its constituent amino acids and vitamins, leading to
a lack of Vitamins B12 and B9 for energy production, detoxification
or neurotransmitters. Or perhaps a history of repeated courses of
antibiotics has left the microbiome—the bacterial community in the
digestive system—lacking key players, which can cause a variety of
digestive issues including IBS.

Along this journey I have come to strongly believe in the body's
ability to heal when provided the building blocks it needs. In your
battle with cancer, you are keenly aware of your body's need. Hello
fatigue, nausea and other symptoms. However, I would venture to
guess that you have not been advised in ways to incorporate food and
other resources to support your body in this battle.

The sad reality is that most doctors barely get any nutritional
training while in medical school. Many doctors want to see evidence-
based information—scientific studies—to support the importance of
food. Yet there is no money available to fund studies that do not result
in a patented return on investment. Real food, as grown in nature,
can't be patented. I have interviewed a wide range of cancer patients
and only one received any guidance for how to nourish her body. The
others noted that none of their doctors ever told them that food might
make a difference in their recovery or resisting recurrence of cancer.
Has that been your experience, too?

Most of the medical community seems to consider food to be
inconsequential to the treatment of disease. Yet there is clear
evidence[1] that inflammation is a major component in the development and spread of cancer. These inflammatory mechanisms are
fueled by our diet.

Beyond wanting to feel better as you navigate this journey, there is a lot more to you than the cancer, whatever its size. Your oncologist is focused solely on the cancer. Sadly, there is usually collateral damage in war. Though radiation may be very specifically targeted, like a guided missile, there is still damage to outer tissue, and chemotherapy effects all the surrounding terrain, as can surgery. My goal is to help you support the cells in your body that aren't directly involved with the tumor or tumors, so that they aren't damaged or lost in the battle.

I'm glad you—or someone who cares about you—have recognized that there must be a better way! Let's start with food and then we will explore how your mind and spirit are also integral players in the process.

Put into Action

Who is on your team for your cancer journey? You have an oncologist and medical team, but who else is supporting you? Of the cancer patients I interviewed, those who had a team around them, both professionals and friends or family, had a smoother journey. I will offer some ideas for your team members, but ultimately you decide who you need. Whether you create a written list or hold one in your head, I encourage you to make note of your team.

Why Do You Eat?

Do you eat to live or live to eat? The answer may be influenced by your culture or your personal tastes and priorities. It may even vary at different times in your life. With the wide variety of food, including its many textures and flavors, it is easy to slip into the "live to eat" mindset. Your body, however, is geared for you to *eat to live*.

Have you ever driven a sports car? It's exhilarating to feel its power enveloping you. The roar of the engine. The speed with which you can accelerate. The smoothness of its movement as you turn the wheel. Sitting at a stop light, you can feel it almost dancing in its readiness to leap forward when the light changes and you press the gas pedal.

What enables that sports car to function as it does? Beyond the design of the body and mechanics, that car demands high octane fuel. You wouldn't put regular gasoline in the tank and expect it to function at its best. You wouldn't have the same power available to respond.

Your body is the same. It is fueled by the food you eat, by way of a very intricate system of digestion.

Beyond *what* you eat, the *way* you eat can significantly affect how your body uses the food. These days it's not unusual to see people eating on the run. It may start with gulping down a cup of coffee and chomping on a pastry as you run out the door in the morning, or pulling in to a fast-food place to grab something quick between meetings later in the day.

Have you ever stopped to think about what is happening to that food once it gets inside your body? First thing's first: let's start with a brief tour through your digestive system, since you may not be aware of all the details. We usually think of our mouths as the place where digestion starts, but it actually begins with our senses—primarily sight and smell. We call this the "cephalic phase of digestion," where you see food and smell the aroma (think about the smell of popcorn in a movie theater). This step attracts you to the food and begins the secretion of saliva and digestive enzymes in your mouth.

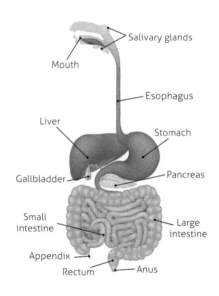

Source: Adobe Stock

THE CEPHALIC PHASE IS USUALLY FOLLOWED BY A BITE OF FOOD entering your mouth, where it is tasted, chewed and swallowed. Sliding down your esophagus, that food arrives in your stomach where it meets a highly acidic environment that helps break it down.

When nearly liquified, your food (now called *chyme*) passes into the small intestine where most of the absorption of nutrients occurs. Depending on what macronutrient components are in your food—carbohydrates, proteins or fats—digestion is accomplished in different parts of the system. Carbohydrates are mostly digested by the time they leave your stomach, while protein digestion starts in the stomach and is completed in the small intestine, and fat digestion doesn't even start until it arrives in your small intestine and is combined with bile from your gall bladder.

The small intestine is about twenty feet long. The inside of your small intestine looks like a strip of shag rug turned inside out. The villi and microvilli (the shag), which line its length, maximize the surface area that supports digestion and absorption of nutrients into your blood stream. Once in the blood, they are delivered to your cells.

Finally, the waste and unabsorbed fiber moves into the large intestine or colon. Here the water and electrolytes are absorbed, leaving a more solid waste product to be eliminated into the toilet. The time between taking a bite and eliminating the waste is called transit time and it averages about fifty-three hours. If it moves too quickly through the intestines, your body isn't absorbing the nutrients; and moving too slowly is constipation. That can allow reabsorption of toxins your body it trying to eliminate, as well as potential damage to the colon.

Physiologically, this whole digestive process is part of the parasympathetic nervous system—also called the "rest and digest" activation. These two functions go together. It's not "*run* and digest."

When you eat on the run, you are not offering your body the opportunity to "rest and digest" but are instead putting it in the opposite position of "fight or flight." Digestion is severely hampered when you are highly stressed, both from your thought processes and the tendency to gulp food without chewing sufficiently.

You don't need to actually be running to interfere with digestion. I had a client who was the mother of four young children. Her husband traveled often, and she was often managing mealtimes on her own, usually eating bites from a plate on the kitchen counter in between answering her children's requests. When I explained that she was functioning in "fight or flight" activation and her body shut off digestive secretions in that mode, she began making changes.

If you are currently in cancer treatment, what do you observe about your digestive system? Is your cephalic phase keyed to the look and smell of food in a way that attracts you, or does it actually repel you from food? I spoke with many who experienced a change in taste, which made it much harder to view food with interest.

Chef Rebecca Katz, author of *The Cancer-Fighting Kitchen*, recommends using small amounts of maple syrup, lemon or lime juice, or sea salt to counter the effects of chemo mouth. She found that when foods taste metallic, a few drops of maple syrup can help. Foods tasting too sweet can be moderated with drops of lemon or lime juice, as can overly salty foods. And if it tastes like cardboard, add a little sea salt.

And what about after you swallow? Does food not feel right in your stomach or down in your belly, where your small intestines and colon are? Are you experiencing diarrhea or constipation, or perhaps a swing from one to another? All of these are signs that digestion is distressed and could use some support.

Here are my foundational guidelines for adding a little more "rest" to a meal and boosting your digestive process:

- Sit down. Seriously. Don't grab your food and head to the next activity. Give yourself a break and take a seat to enjoy even a small meal. And don't rush off after you finish the meal. Relax for a few minutes.

- Pause ... take five deep breaths before you start eating, pausing each time you inhale before exhaling slowly. This practice helps to shift you into parasympathetic activation. It is a simple way to prepare for digestion and to reduce your stress levels. If you find yourself stressed during the day, plan times to just stop, close your eyes, and breathe deeply.
- Chew. When you take a bite, chew more than you usually would. "Chomp-chomp-swallow" is not chewing for good digestion and is actually one of the primary causes of digestive distress! Chewing is the only part of the process you can control, and it provides important mechanical and chemical preparation of your food for the next stage. Practice *really* chewing—until your food is nearly liquified before you swallow. Start with a basic approach of ten chews for soft food and twenty for meats and dense foods. Challenging, I know. Think of it like chewing gum. You will have the urge to swallow after just a few chews but move the food to your cheek while you swallow saliva, and then continue chewing. Not only will your digestion be greatly improved, but you may find yourself satisfied with less food.
- Put your utensil down between bites. This keeps you from habitually rushing to put the next bite in your mouth. If you are eating finger foods or a sandwich, put it down between bites as well.
- Still finding a slower pace challenging? Try holding your utensil in your non-dominant hand. If you are right-handed, use the fork or spoon in your left hand which will make you focus more on the process of eating, thus slowing you down.

Slowing your pace to ensure you are in the "rest and digest" mode will not only support better digestion downstream but will also give your body time to register when it is full. During a meal, your body releases a hormone called cholecystokinin (CCK) which signals your brain that you are full. CCK is generally released about fifteen-to-twenty minutes after you start eating. Eating too fast can set the stage for overeating. Slow down and give your body the opportunity to gauge the volume of your meal and digest it well.

Though you can't control every aspect of digestion, you do have the ability to support your body's use of the food you consume by following these simple guidelines. Old habits may seem hard to change, but I'm hoping that the story of my client will demonstrate that knowledge can motivate different choices. What will you change first?

Put into Action

Experiment with the steps I have recommended during your next several meals. How difficult was it to chew a lot before you swallowed? It may take some practice, but it will make a difference for your digestion if you make the effort. Did you find it hard to sit and slow down as you ate? This too, may take some practice, and I know your body will benefit as you slow the meal process.

The Elephant in The Room

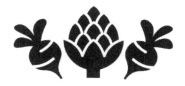

We've explored the reason for eating and how our digestive system works. I think it is important that we also address the elephant in the room - the sugar content of your food.

If you have spent time in a cancer treatment center, especially for infusions, I'm sure that you have seen what my friend reported. She told me that in an effort to support the patients in maintaining their weight, the staff offers them snacks such as sandwiches, granola bars, cookies or candy. Is this what you have seen, too? The problem? These "foods" are loaded with sugar or ingredients that turn quickly to sugar in the body—and, as I explain below, sugar feeds cancer.

Many programs include meeting with a nutritionist in preparation for or during treatment. The consensus of what I heard in my interviews with patients who met with a nutritionist was that the focus was on eating to maintain weight, and if that included donuts and ice cream, that was fine. Was that your experience too?

While maintaining your weight during treatment is important, there are ways to do so that don't compromise other processes in your body. If this is a concern for you, I cover it in Chapter 12. First, let me share with you why sugar (or glucose) works against you, both in normal physiology and in your battle with cancer. Your medical team is primarily focused on the cancer, and the means used to battle that cancer can be very hard on the rest of your body as well. Sugar, though a delight on your tongue, has some very detrimental effects in your body:

- High glucose levels in your blood stream cause inflammation[1] in the lining of the arteries to your heart, which can set off a series of processes that increase your risk of stroke or heart attack.
- High glucose levels damage the kidney's very sensitive filtration system.
- Proteins incorporate sugar from the blood stream into their structure which speeds up the aging of tissue and skin, causing wrinkles.
- Sugar or glucose can rewire the brain's pathways contributing to higher incidence of depression.
- High glucose levels impair blood flow and can lead to dehydration as the kidneys produce more urine in an effort to clear the excess glucose.
- Malignant cells favor glucose for anaerobic energy production.

Cancer cells are different from the normal cells in your body. Picture a community living in an apartment complex. The buildings are well-maintained with grass, trees, and gardens in the common spaces. The families living in this community come from very different backgrounds and work in different ways each day, and they visit with each other while the children play outside and interact with each other in passing. These families could be equated to tissues and organs—groups of individual cells that have a common purpose—living in the community of the body. Each has a particular purpose, but all enjoy oxygen, energy from a variety of sources and connection with other cells. And they are all known by the community police force—the immune system—that monitors the families and their cells to ensure they are safe and living (producing energy) efficiently.

But there is a recluse in the community. This family of cells doesn't communicate with those around it and avoids the oxygen it would get from being outside with others. It hides itself from the community police force and craves only glucose, though it doesn't produce energy efficiently as the others in the community do.

This recluse is cancer. Though part of your body, it stays separate. While normal cells can efficiently produce energy from a variety of sources using aerobic respiration, cancer cells are metabolically damaged.[2] They avoid oxygen and favor glucose for anaerobic energy production which produces significantly less energy along with lactic acid and carbon needed for rapid cell growth. The lactic acid creates a smokescreen to help the cancer hide from your body's normal immune response.

Some of your body's immune cells act like PacMan from the old video game, engulfing and gobbling up invaders. While PacMan was fueled by pellets he consumed as he moved through the game, our white blood cells are energized by Vitamin C. Consuming foods with lots of sugar, or grain-based foods like breads, crackers, pasta, cookies, and cakes, quickly raises the level of glucose in your blood stream. This limits the amount of Vitamin C that can enter your white blood cells and can reduce their activity by up to 75%.[3] Not only does reduced Vitamin C limit your white blood cells' effectiveness, their ability to reproduce is also limited. High glucose levels cause your army to dwindle. A caution, lest you assume from what I am sharing that you need more Vitamin C and reach for a glass of orange juice. Please press "pause" on that thought and I will explain more in Chapter 7.

Cancer treatment can deplete your energy levels, which is another reason that you might reach for a sugary snack or drink. Fatigue can be caused by many factors in your body—changes in protein and hormone levels linked to inflammation, a build-up of cellular waste that requires cleanup and repair, changes in activity level, higher toxicity that your body is trying to clear, and changes in blood counts and electrolytes. All of these require added energy to be directed to these functions, which reduce what is available to you for everyday activities.

You now know how cancer cells use glucose, but what about your normal cells? They may use glucose or fat interchangeably, but glucose tends to be more plentiful in the average diet. Normal cells convert glucose to ATP (Adenosine Triphosphate—the energy currency of your body) in their mitochondria. You could picture it like the engine room of an old steamship. Coal is shoveled into the furnace to keep the fire burning as consistently as possible. When the coal supply is depleted, the ship slows down, and more coal is loaded aboard. This works steadily along the route to keep the ship moving.

But what if a new supply of coal is delivered multiple times in the day, before the old supply is depleted? The engine room would have piles of coal encroaching on all the areas where the enginemen need to work, and potentially would limit their ability to get the coal into the furnace. This could cause the steamship's fire to go out and the ship to founder on its journey, despite having a plentiful supply of coal.

Likewise, your mitochondria can get so crowded with glucose supply that they are not able to function efficiently. Your non-cancer cells can struggle for energy while the cancer in your body is finding just what it needs to fuel its growth. Would you agree this is not a good situation?

As I have mentioned, your medical team is likely more focused on your maintaining weight, and not as concerned about the physiological effects of sugar consumption. So, it's up to you to use this information to guide your choices on a daily basis in order to minimize the sugar you supply to cancer cells.

Put into Action

What has been your norm up to this point? How prominent are sugar sources in your pantry and refrigerator? What will be the first change you will make? If your doctor is concerned about your weight, you have probably been encouraged to eat or drink anything that is high in calories. Perhaps what I have shared in this chapter is disturbing to you—it might even make you feel that you are caught between a rock and a hard place. I have provided guidance in Chapter 10 on how to maintain or gain weight in a healthful manner.

The Nutrition of Color

PICTURE IN YOUR MIND A BUSY DAY WHEN YOU HAD appointments scheduled and you needed to be in several places around town. When hunger struck you pulled into the nearest fast-food joint. Maybe you chose to go inside and sit down for a quick bite, but more likely you went through the drive-through to grab something to munch on as you headed to your next objective.

As you unwrapped the food, what colors were in front of you? Condiments don't count. Was the packaging more colorful than the food?

Did your meal have visual appeal, or was it simply a collection of foods that would fill your stomach with a taste you liked?

Did you eat the colors of the rainbow? Most likely, the answer is no.

Why does it matter? Because the color of your food is an indicator of the nutrients that it contains. That is the natural colors in food, not the artificial colors that are often added. Contrary to popular opinion, nutrients are the reason you eat. At least, that is what your body is seeking when it calls for food. Your body needs you to eat for it to live.

Add some color and what do you gain? Nutrients...energy...life! Let's look at what the colors represent for your body.

Put some **green** on your plate—whether raw or cooked, the darker the better—and you will be supporting improved eye health and up-regulating detox enzymes in your liver. This is important when your body is receiving a lot of medication. Options could include leafy greens, cucumber, broccoli, green beans, zucchini, kiwi, or avocado. Green vegetables and fruits provide perhaps the widest range of vitamins and minerals including a great source of calcium, iron, potassium, and folate.

Another color you could add to your plate is **blue** or **purple**, which will greatly increase your antioxidant support, fight inflammation in your circulatory system, boost your immune system, and improve the health of your skin. All of these are important for supporting your body in the battle with cancer. By incorporating foods like blueberries, blackberries, red cabbage, or eggplant, you will be supporting your body with added Vitamin C, potassium, and folate.

Besides green, blue, and purple, another color that stands out when you scan the produce department display is **red**. There are many options from which to choose. Perhaps first in mind is an apple, along with cherries, strawberries, pomegranate, cranberries, and raspberries in the fruit section, and tomatoes, red peppers, rhubarb, beets, and radishes among the vegetables. The lycopene, quercetin, anthocyanin, and Vitamin C these foods provide for your body promote heart health and reduce inflammation, reducing your risk of stroke and macular degeneration. These are definitely needed by your body.

Closely related to the red foods are the **orange** and **yellow** ones. Your first thoughts in this category are likely the familiar orange and lemon, but there are more. Carrots, sweet potatoes, pumpkin, orange and yellow peppers, pineapples, peaches, and spaghetti squash are other candidates that come to mind.

Are you wondering why I left corn out of the list in the yellow category? Many of us grew up thinking corn was a vegetable but—

surprise!—it is actually a grain and a prominent source of starch (think "sugar") in your body. I would recommend focusing on other vegetables to increase your nutrient value.

What nutrients do you gain from eating orange and yellow produce? There are many, including beta-carotene, potassium, and Vitamins A and C. You've no doubt heard from childhood that beta-carotene supports eye and skin health, and these vegetables and fruits also provide electrolytes and anti-inflammatory compounds. Winning additions to support the cells in your body!

Now lest you think I'm completely omitting a color category, I agree that **white** is a color in vegetables and fruit with some benefit. Cauliflower, onions, and potatoes probably come to mind, yet there are many other candidates. When you look past the skin color you find pears, leeks, jicama, parsnips, shallots, and kohlrabi are white. White fruits and vegetables provide sulfur compounds associated with strong bones and healthy blood vessels, plus the antioxidant compound quercetin, and a wealth of selenium, potassium, riboflavin, and niacin. All of these help to maintain healthy blood cells, lower blood cholesterol levels, and reduce free radical damage.

PHYTONUTRIENTS IN FRUIT & VEGETABLE COLORS

COLOR	INCLUDES	PHYTONUTRIENTS	BENEFITS
Red	Apples, tomatoes, pomagranate, cherries, watermelon, radish, raspberries	Lycopene, Elagic acid, Quercetin, Hesperidin, Anthocyanidins	Supports urinary tract, prostate, and DNA health. Counters heart disease risks.
Green	Broccoli, lettuce, kale, kiwi, honeydew, spinach, avocado, cucumber	Lutein/Zeaxanthin, EGCG, Indoles, Sulphoraphane, Isothiocyanates	Supports eye, cell, and lung health, and arterial and liver function. Helps wound healing.
Blue/Purple	Cabbage, blueberry, fig, grape, plum, eggplant, purple cabbage, blackberry	Resveratrol, Anthocyanidins, Phenolics, Flavanoids	Benefits heart, brain, artery, bone, and cognitive health. Fights cancer and free radical damage.
Yellow/Orange	Lemon, orange, sweet potato, squash, carrot, papaya, peach, pineapple, peppers	Alpha-carotenes, Beta-carotenes, Lutein/Zeaxanthin, Hesperidin	Benefits eye health and immune function. Supports healthy growth and development.
White	Cauliflower, onion, leek, pear, banana, jicama, parsnips, mushrooms, garlic	Allicin, Quercetin, EGCG, Indoles, Glucosinolates	Supports healthy bones and circulatory system. Fights heart disease and cancer.

WHERE DO YOU FIND THE MOST CONSISTENT SOURCE OF FOOD colors in your grocery store? That's right—the produce section! Oh, there are lots of colors up and down the aisles, but they are primarily on the packaging. The foods in the package contain artificial colors that can present a whole new set of challenges for your body.

You can greatly increase both the variety and the nutrition in your meals by swapping out bland-colored, processed foods in favor of more colorful vegetables and fruits. Your senses will be both stimulated and nourished by boosting the color scheme on your plate, and your body will benefit from the added fiber and energy provided by these lively foods.

I have had clients who struggled with lack of appetite and metallic taste that made it a challenge to eat what their body needed. One asked about taking a multi-vitamin to make up the difference and I shared with her the importance of selecting quality brands. The majority of multi-vitamins available include synthetic ingredients that the body can't use effectively. What is key for nutrition is both consuming and absorbing the nutrients.

Capsules of freeze-dried fruits and vegetables are available that the body will recognize and use their nutrients. One of the cancer patients that I interviewed reported that her cravings for sugar were reduced when she included these in her daily support. If you find it challenging to eat a variety of fruit and vegetables to nourish your body, you may want to visit my book portal for further information on how to access these quality supplements.

The color of your food provides so much more than visual appeal. It is vital for nutrient density, provided the color does not come from artificial sources. There's no substitute for the produce that grows on plants and trees. If you must seek support in capsule form, be sure that it is sourced from whole food so that your body has a lifeline from nature.

Put into Action

- Observe the food you are eating and take note of the colors on your plate.
- What do you see the most?
- What colors are missing?
- Of the missing colors, pick one to add to your meals.
- You could choose a vegetable from the chart above or explore the produce section to find an option.
- Not sure how to prepare it? An online search for "whole food recipe (name of the vegetable you chose)" and review the options.

Eat Foods in The Right Order

We have already talked about the effect that sugar can have on your body and cancer cells. If you have ever watched an episode of *Sesame Street*, you could imagine that sugar makes cancer cells as excited as the Cookie Monster with a plate of cookies. Those cells are metabolically damaged and have a huge hunger for sugar (glucose), to provide lactic acid that disguises their presence and carbon for rapid growth. Part of the strategy for fighting cancer is limiting its fuel source, which can not only be done through the choices you make regarding food, but also the order in which you eat your food.

We all have patterns in the way we eat, which are usually reflected in the way food is served at a restaurant. Yet, these patterns often set us up for a higher glucose spike that could feed cancer cells or generally contribute to damage in our bodies that leads to disease. When you begin your meal with grain- or flour-based foods (bread or chips at a restaurant) or a bowl of cereal for breakfast, those foods turn quickly into glucose causing a quick rise in your blood sugar. This spike of glucose prompts the release of insulin to bring the levels down. When the foods you eat cause repeated spikes of glucose and insulin release throughout the day, your cells will likely reduce their receptivity to insulin (causing insulin resistance), resulting in more storage of glucose as fat.

You may be wondering how fruit plays into this situation? Some believe that the fructose from fruit is more natural and therefore "healthier," yet that really isn't the case. Fructose must be processed in the liver before it is released into the body, and that can cause added strain on the liver. I wouldn't say completely eliminate fruit but consider it another sugar source in your diet. One recommendation I always share with my clients is to eliminate fruit juice and use very little fruit in their smoothies. When fruit is juiced, all the fiber is removed and what you have left is the water and fructose—essentially, a sugar infusion. If you know someone with diabetes, they would confirm to you that when their sugar drops to a low level, they drink orange juice to raise their blood glucose quickly. It meets their need at the time, but is not a practice I would recommend regularly. Smoothies that primarily contain fruit are similar to sugar-laden beverages. A better approach for smoothies would be to use mostly vegetables and just a little fruit (apple, berries or half a banana) to sweeten the taste.

Anyone with a diagnosis of diabetes is familiar with monitoring their blood sugar levels and modifying the way they eat to reduce the spikes or high curves after eating particular foods. But it's not all about the glucose in foods. Fat, fiber, fructose, and insulin also influence how high the curve goes. The good news? You don't have to master all the nutritional details. Instead, focus on putting a few key hacks into action and your glucose curve will be significantly reduced.

CONSUME FOODS IN THIS ORDER

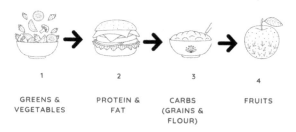

1	2	3	4
GREENS & VEGETABLES	PROTEIN & FAT	CARBS (GRAINS & FLOUR)	FRUITS

Greens and Vegetables

Start your meals with a small bowl of greens—Romaine, Spinach, Chard, and Butter lettuce are just a few of the options. Eating a packed cup of these greens drizzled with olive oil and a dash of salt and pepper for flavor will lay a mat of fiber in your stomach that will slow the digestion of foods you eat after the greens.

Think of your kitchen sink. When you place a rubber mat or even a plate in the bottom of the sink over the drain, it slows the flow of water and other items down the drain. This small bowl of greens will do the same. Your stomach acid will work on the greens and release them into your small intestines, while slowing the flow of other foods that are more likely to increase your glucose curve.

To clarify, when I say "greens" I am referring to what you may think of as salad greens. They are less dense and easily eaten to provide the benefit of the mat in your stomach. You can change up your greens, mixing in spring greens, arugula, even mustard or turnip greens. Not accustomed to eating them? Start with romaine, butter lettuce, or spinach for a simpler flavor. Then explore other choices as you become more accustomed to the practice.

Greens are recommended for creating the mat to balance the glucose curve because they are easier to chew and consume at the beginning of a meal. I hope you have other vegetables in your meal—remember, they are the way you add color and nutrients. You can also eat a portion of those first after your greens, followed by the protein and fat.

Protein and Fats

Protein and fats provide not only essential nutritional components for your body, but are also digested more slowly and, therefore, help you feel full longer. Eating meat or other sources of protein and fat will lower the effect of grain-based foods eaten at the end of the meal.[4] I always recommend combining a protein or fat source with greens and vegetables or carbohydrates, whether for a meal or a snack, to avoid feeling hungry again shortly after you have eaten.

Carbohydrates

It's best to wait until later in your meal to eat the foods made from grains or flour because those quickly convert to glucose (sugar) in your system. By eating the greens and vegetables (fiber), protein and fat first, your body won't experience the quick spike in blood sugar that is caused by carbs eaten early in the meal.[5] There is also a bonus benefit in the likelihood that you will feel full sooner and not eat as many carbs.

Fruit

Likewise, I recommend saving fruit for last because it, too, will raise your blood sugar and we want to keep it as steady as possible. As I mentioned before, the sugar we get from fruit is fructose. Fructose cannot be used directly by your cells for energy as glucose can, because it must first be converted into usable forms by the liver. High levels of fructose, including what is consumed as high fructose corn syrup in processed foods and agave syrup, affect the body's metabolism and prompt weight gain.

Consume fruit after you eat protein or fat, ideally as the "dessert" for your meal. If you like to eat fruit for a snack, I suggest pairing it with almond butter or another unsweetened nut butter or hummus to provide the protein and fat to slow the spike in blood sugar.

What might this look like for your meal? If you were eating spaghetti for dinner, what would you start with to lay the mat in your stomach? Greens. Then you need to consider what your spaghetti normally looks like. Are you a minimalist who likes pasta with sauce? In that case, I would recommend you add a source of protein on the side—perhaps a piece of chicken or other meat—to eat after the greens and before you eat the spaghetti. If you like a meat sauce, make it a really chunky meat sauce served over less pasta. Even better, eat a vegetable after your greens and before you eat the spaghetti.

What's for Breakfast?

Did you grow up eating a bowl of cereal for breakfast most mornings? I did. No matter what the front of the box says, the cereal inside has been highly processed to remove fiber and will cause a quick spike in blood sugar that will prompt your body to store fat and will send the cancer cells into a tizzy.

Breakfast is the meal most likely to cause a significant spike in blood sugar and insulin because it is typically laden with grains and sugar. This meal in which you "break the fast" is key for setting up your metabolism for the day. When you start your day with a big surge in glucose, your body will be geared for storing fat and your cells will suffer, except of course for the cancer cells.

What is your normal breakfast? I have had clients who thought they were making a better choice by switching from breakfast cereal to granola or muesli, but these still cause a spike in blood sugar. Other clients prefer to have a piece of toast with coffee in the morning, which can be fine, depending on what is on the toast. A plain piece of toast will cause a significant spike, as will toast spread with jam or jelly. But if you spread your toast with unsweetened almond butter or avocado—sources of protein and fat—the blood glucose spike is reduced. A simple change can make a big difference!

Likewise, trading your fruit smoothie for eggs or an omelet and some vegetables will flatten your curve and give your body some valuable protein for better function. You could even add some meat, but I would suggest you avoid sausage, as most of these have unknown ingredients and chemical preservatives that could work against you.

It warrants repeating here: fruit juices, though they have been considered breakfast beverages for decades, act like sugar infusions in your body. Because they are in liquid form, little digestion is needed in the stomach and the juice is quickly absorbed into the blood stream. Hence, I do not recommend drinking fruit juices, but only eating whole fruit with its fiber intact at the end of your meal.

Eat and Then Move

Food fuels many processes in your body and supplies energy for your muscles to move. Movement is a great way to use up blood sugar spikes that may occur with a meal or a snack. Perhaps pause long enough after your meal to clean up the dishes and then move. And I'm not recommending that you move to a level that causes you to sweat, but simply take a walk around the block, walk up and down a couple flights of stairs, or turn on a song and do a little dance. Not only will this movement help to flatten the blood sugar curve but it will also lift your mood. It's a win, win!

Put into Action

If you realized as you read this chapter that your breakfast is focused more on carbohydrates, change it up. For the next three mornings, eat a breakfast that is focused on protein, and observe how your body responds. I'm confident that you will notice an improvement in the way you feel, so continue to eat a protein-focused breakfast to reduce your blood sugar level.

Are Your Beverages Hydrating?

ONE OF THE MOST INSIDIOUS SOURCES OF CALORIES IS THE beverages that we drink so casually each day. Those who log their food intake may be fastidious about writing down every food eaten, but it is not unusual to overlook the beverages they drink.

Has your oncologist encouraged you to keep your weight up during treatment? If so, you were given carte blanche permission to eat whatever appealed to you—donuts, ice cream, milkshake, whatever. Unfortunately, the first things that come to mind for taste and weight gain are those loaded with sugar, and we have already talked about how that is ultimately working against you.

Empty Calories

It is so very common for people to consume high-calorie sugar infusions daily. These have many names. Let's review some of the potential candidates:

EMPTY CALORIES

ITEM	CALORIES	GRAMS OF SUGAR	OTHER DETAILS
Starbuck's Grande White Chocolate Mocha ™	410	67 (nearly 17 teaspoons!)	
McCafe ®Medium Iced Mocha	340	43 (nearly 11 teaspoons!)	
Medium Fast-Food Soda	210 (average)	58	and a free refill!
Monster Energy XXL	300	81 (20 teaspoons or 7 tablespoons!)	Plus the caffeine equal to 3 cups of coffee
Gatorade Frost Glacier Cherry	140	34 (8.5 teaspoons!)	
Burger King Strawberry Shake	610	90 (22.5 teaspoons!)	Not ONE strawberry

These selections are just a sampling of what is available, and they are loaded with enough sugar to cause a significant spike in your blood sugar—followed by a crash in energy when your body responds with insulin. Not only that, but their liquid form enables that sugar spike to happen much faster than if it was consumed in solid food that requires digestion first. Why is this a problem? Because each sugar spike prompts release of insulin to manage the blood sugar, and repetitive spikes raise the levels of insulin that circulate in the blood. Elevated insulin can cause issues with your hormones, cardiovascular system, and more.

Between the sugar content and the liquid form, your body doesn't register beverages in the same way as the food you eat. You may actually be consuming 1,000 additional calories or more without realizing it because what we drink doesn't seem to fill us up in the same way.

Now, you may be thinking that you are off the hook if you regularly choose sugar-free beverages, most of which have artificial sweeteners. Many people feel that they are countering the challenges of sugar by opting for beverages made with the ingredients of those little blue, pink or yellow packets. However, there are many concerns about the long-term effects of artificial sweeteners, and I, personally, avoid them.

Chemical Concoction

You may have a long history of enjoying diet drinks without much thought to the side effects of the chemicals that sweeten them. Unless you explore holistic health resources, you may not hear anyone raise questions about their safety. But there are numerous studies that reveal concerns.

First of all, products with aspartame, acesulfame-K, sucralose or saccharin, have been repeatedly shown to promote weight gain.[6] What?! This is due to normal physiology that causes your body to expect an influx of energy with sweet tasting food or beverage. In the absence of that expected energy, your body raises your hunger level, propelling you to eat more.

Not a problem, you may be thinking, since your doctor wants you to eat to maintain your weight during treatment. Yet there are other negative effects that are more concerning.

These include a greater risk of developing Type 2 diabetes, metabolic syndrome[7], depression[8], and digestive issues[9] that lead to malabsorption and set you up for chronic disease—as though cancer[10] wasn't enough. I strongly recommend that you steer clear of those artificial sweeteners.

What is the primary reason that you are drinking liquids?

Hydration

You drink liquids for the moisture they offer. Your body is 65% water, and water is involved in most every function of the organs and systems inside.

Everyday activities—including talking, breathing, sweating that accompanies exercise, and elimination—cause the loss of water, which must be replenished.

What are the common symptoms of dehydration? I'm sure your first thought was thirst or dry mouth, which are well known. There are other symptoms that you may not automatically associate with dehydration, including dry skin, fatigue, headache, dizziness, and dark urine.

When you have a headache, you don't likely think of chugging a tall glass of water—at least not without an aspirin involved. Yet, you may be very surprised to find that simply drinking the water and waiting five to ten minutes will often bring relief.

So, what do you normally drink? What are the ingredients, and are they supporting hydration, or are they hindering it? If your drink incorporates sugar or chemicals, as I mentioned above, your body does not recognize it as a hydration source.

If coffee is a go-to beverage, you may be disappointed to hear that it can dehydrate you, even if you drink it black. My recommendation would be to start with a glass of water first thing to hydrate your body after sleep and then drink your coffee.

Your body needs W.A.T.E.R. The simpler, the better. You can infuse the water with tea leaves, or with fruit slices and herbs as you would find in infused water recipes; but adding more ingredients than these tends to make your beverage more likely to **de**hydrate rather than hydrate.

The next time you are beginning to feel the signs of dehydration, try a cleaner alternative that your body will use and appreciate. If you don't like the taste of the water in your area, I recommend getting a filtration system that will remove the chemicals and minerals that influence its flavor. I don't recommend using bottled water regularly because studies have shown that it contains microplastics from the bottles, along with chemicals that leech into the water when the bottles are stored long term or exposed to high or very low heat.

Mineral Water

One form of water that we Americans don't often consider is mineral water (think "Perrier" or "sparkling water"). When I lived in Europe, it was very common to have a bottle of mineral water on the table when we sat down at a restaurant, as opposed to the American practice of serving glasses of water. Though I didn't particularly like its taste at first, I found that I grew accustomed to it, and realized that it was more effective at satisfying thirst than plain water, thanks to the higher mineral content. Why not try it for yourself?

Infused Waters

Do you struggle with drinking water because it seems boring? You aren't alone! Have you tried infused water? The most common way of infusing water is the slice of lemon that is served with your water or iced tea at many restaurants. It's a start, and there are so many other possibilities, such as:

- **Pineapple and Mint**. Put two spears of fresh pineapple and a sprig of fresh mint into a quart-sized Mason jar and fill with water. Put a lid on and refrigerate overnight. Strain and enjoy!
- **Blueberry, Orange, and Basil.** Put two slices of a peeled orange, ten-to-fifteen squeezed blueberries, and six torn basil leaves into a two-quart pitcher and top with water. Let sit and diffuse for several hours before straining to serve.
- **Cucumber, Lemon, and Cilantro**. Peel and slice ½ a lemon and combine it with a few sprigs of cilantro and a sliced cucumber in a two-quart pitcher. Fill the pitcher with water and refrigerate overnight. Strain and enjoy the refreshing, clean taste.

Side note: many of my clients find they enjoy lemon or lime in their water, both for the flavor and the added electrolyte benefit. Because agricultural pesticides can be trapped in the oils on the skin of citrus, I recommend that you squeeze the juice into your water but not drop the squeezed rind into your glass. By doing so, you may have pesticides seeping into the water that you will drink. We don't need those chemicals absorbed into our bodies along with our hydration.

There are many other possible combinations for infused waters. My favorite source of ideas is found at infusedwaters.com—give these a try and start hydrating your body with flavor that your mouth will enjoy.

Put into Action

What do you normally drink through the day? Of the total cups or glasses you drink, how many glasses were water? If less than three-quarters are water, I encourage you to swap one each day for a glass of water, either plain or infused. You can upgrade the benefits of your beverages one glass at a time.

What's Old Is New Again

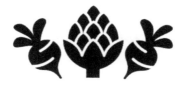

Chicken soup isn't just good for the soul, it has many benefits for the body as well. Made with chicken bone broth, it is full of nutrients that are easy to absorb, offers rich flavors and boosts healing for your digestive system and other tissue.

Traditional cultures and trained chefs have used bone broth for ages, and not all old practices are outdated. It began hundreds of years ago as a way to use every part of an animal. For the past century, science has shown repeatedly that the nutrients in bone broth are beneficial to many areas of the body.[11]

You may have heard different terms such as broth, stock and bone broth. There are slight differences between these, so let me outline those to ensure that what I'm addressing is what you are thinking.

Broth is typically made with meat and a small amount of bone, simmering them for a relatively short time of one-to-two hours. This produces a thin liquid with a light flavor that is rich in protein.

Stock is generally made with roasted bones and a small amount of meat that still adheres to them. It is simmered for about three-to-four hours which produces a liquid that is rich in minerals and gelatin.

Bone broth, which is what I'm going to discuss in this chapter, is also made with roasted bones and a small amount of meat, but it is simmered for twenty-four hours or longer in order to remove the maximum minerals and nutrients, along with gelatin and collagen. Modern pressure cookers can significantly reduce the time required to make bone broth.

In addition to the minerals, gelatin, and collagen, bone broth provides a number of amino acids that are key to its benefits for the body. These include **Proline, Glycine, Arginine** and **Glutamine**. When you read about nutrients, you have probably come across the terms "essential" and "non-essential." Essential nutrients are ones that we must consume through our food because they cannot be made in the body. Though the four amino acids mentioned above are not normally considered "essential," if your health is compromised, your body is probably not able to effectively make what is needed.

Why are these amino acids so important? I'm providing an overview, but feel free to skip these paragraphs if it is too much for you. You don't have to understand the science to benefit from consuming bone broth.

Proline and hydroxyproline are used in building collagen, which is a key component in connective tissue for bone, skin, muscles, tendon, and cartilage. It helps make tissue strong, resilient, and able to withstand stretching. Collagen also keeps your arteries pliable so that blood can circulate without isn't hindrance.

Glycine is the simplest of amino acids that is used in myriad ways. It is involved in the synthesis of RNA and DNA, which are essential for cellular function, and glutathione, which is the body's master antioxidant. Glycine also supports liver function, blood sugar regulation, and the gastric acid secretion[12] as well as protecting skeletal muscle from wasting.[13] It's a busy little molecule.

Besides boosting my glycine supply through bone broth, I also use powdered glycine as a sweetener in my hot tea. It's a great way to get the sweet flavor I want without adding detrimental side effects that come with sugar or artificial sweeteners. If you are vegetarian or vegan and do not consume products from animals, you can get these other amino acids from supplements. I am cautious about brands because supplements are not policed and may have poor forms or sources of ingredients that would limit your benefit.

Arginine is another amino acid that works in conjunction with glycine to support kidney function and improve wound healing.

Lastly, bone broth offers an easily absorbed source of **glutamine**. This amino acid has been controversial in cancer treatment. Glutamine is a key building block for restoring the intestinal lining and supporting the immune system. It also can help to stabilize blood glucose levels and build healthy muscles. During prolonged periods of illness, the body will break down muscle tissue to extract glutamine, hence the loss of muscle mass that is common with chronic disease.

Some oncologists are concerned that glutamine can increase the reproduction of tumors. Yet, recent studies have demonstrated benefit from decreased metabolic side effects resulting from cancer treatment and improved patient outcomes.[14] As has been mentioned before, there is a lot more to your body than the cancer. Providing nutrients that support the function of the rest of your body will enable you to withstand the effects of the treatment without being depleted.[15, 16]

According to Dr. Paul S. Anderson, medical director of Anderson Medical Specialty Associates, "The availability of glutamine even in a supplemented person is often too low to do much more than feed the deficient GI [gastrointestinal] cells, so peripheral use is limited with oral doses. The one common exception is glioblastoma multiforme." That's medical speak to say that glutamine supplements provide just enough to nourish the struggling intestinal cells,[17] but not enough to encourage tumor growth, except in the case of glioblastoma multiforme.

In addition to the amino acids, the gelatin in bone broth aids in absorption of the vitamins and minerals it provides. Those whose digestion is challenged by meats often find it far easier to digest if meat is served with a broth-based gravy, cooked in bone broth or eaten after drinking a cup of bone broth. Don't forget that chewing fully, as addressed in Chapter 3, is especially important.

Bone broth has long been recognized as both a nourishing drink and a valuable foundation for cooking. One caution for you: most store-bought stock and broth are not "real" but contain lab-produced meat flavors and monosodium glutamate, which may taste good but are not nourishing. The best bone broth is generally made at home or purchased from reputable vendors. All you need is a large pot, a couple chicken carcasses, water, vegetables and a stove. An Instant Pot can also speed the process.

If you are concerned about consumption of bone broth containing glutamine, I encourage you to discuss it with your oncologist and provide the references I have given in the back of the book for review.

Put into Action

I have included some broth recipes in the Book Portal. Make a batch and drink ½ cup daily.

Read the Labels

THE GREATEST LEVEL OF NUTRITION IS FOUND IN WHOLE OR real foods. But what are whole or real foods? They are defined as "food that is unprocessed and unrefined, or processed and refined as little as possible." Lisa, the blogger from *100 Days of Real Food*, defines real food as no refined grains, no refined or artificial sweeteners, nothing out of a package that contains more than five ingredients, and no deep-fried or fast foods. Basically, food that is more a product of nature than of a factory.

Where do you find these foods? The more refined the food, the longer it will last on the shelf, so the whole or real foods are generally found around the perimeter of the grocery store where you find the perishable foods displayed.

What has been your normal source of foods? Do you generally eat food prepared by a restaurant, or frozen or packaged foods that are quick to cook? You may not have had the habit of spending much time in the kitchen up until this point.

My recommendation is that you begin to explore ways that you can prepare foods that are simple, both in preparation and in ingredients. Foods from restaurants, whether fast food or not, often have a lot of ingredients that you can't track and may be working against your body. An example would be strawberry milkshakes served at most fast-food chains. Have you ever explored their ingredients? You would probably be shocked to discover that there usually are no strawberries in them. The flavor is created by chemical additives with artificial food coloring. Doesn't seem fair, does it?

Likewise, packaged foods are sure to have preservatives and ingredients that are best avoided. I often tell my clients that if a food is packaged so that it can be kept on a shelf or in a vending machine for months without spoiling, it doesn't offer you benefit either. If no self-respecting bacteria would eat it, how would it nourish your body?

A good place to start is in your kitchen. When you open your refrigerator what do you see? Is there fresh produce in the lower drawers, lots of deli meats and cheeses, to-go boxes or storage containers with leftovers from home-prepared meals? Deli meats usually have preservatives and chemicals that do not benefit our bodies, as do foods that we consume at restaurants. Fresh, perishable food is ideal because it has more nutrients and enzymes for your body. I realize that isn't always feasible, depending on your situation, yet it can be a goal to pursue step by step.

And what do you have in your pantry? Lots of boxed mixes for preparing food, crackers and cookies, or canned goods and jars? Though many of these were made from ingredients that were fresh at the beginning of the process, once they are packaged to be kept on a shelf long term, there is little real nutrition to be found in those foods. Pull out a couple of the boxes or jars and look at their nutrition and ingredient labels.

These are usually found together on the same panel of the packaging, with the nutrition label showing the serving size, calories, fat, cholesterol, sodium, carbohydrates and protein included in that serving. The ingredient label shows what is included in the product.

I personally don't rely too heavily on the information provided on the **nutrition label**, as this can be manipulated by the manufacturer. It is interesting to me, though, to look at the **serving size** at the top of that label. If you were to purchase a twenty ounce carbonated beverage and look at its nutrition label, you would likely be surprised to see that it is considered two servings. Listing it this way makes the calorie and carbohydrate levels listed further down the label appear less distressing. Most boxed cereals list ¾ cup as the serving size, but how many people do you know who actually eat that small a serving? I would say twice that is more common, unless you have someone in your house who eats cereal like Jethro on *The Beverly Hillbillies* TV show—poured into a mixing bowl with a quart of milk.

Before you can determine whether a product fits your dietary needs, you may need to do some calculations. What is the portion you actually eat of this food, and what are the modified levels of sodium and carbohydrate components you are consuming?

Besides the serving size, you might notice how much **sodium** is in a serving of the food in the package, modified by the serving size you would actually eat. Sodium is added to food for flavor and preservation and to speed the cooking process. We need sodium in our diet, but not the amount that is normally consumed in a diet of processed foods. Before you eat something that came in a package, think to yourself: how much of a 1,500 milligram daily allowance would this one product fill?

The amount of sodium can reflect the preservatives in the food as well as the speed at which it cooks. Oatmeal is an easy example. Rolled or old-fashioned oats don't have added salt and have more fiber than quick oats, which have added salt and less fiber. Instant oatmeal has even more salt and the least amount of fiber, helping it cook faster. TV dinners are known to have lots of salt in them and relatively little fiber, even when they include vegetables.

Lastly, I suggest that you look at the **carbohydrate** section, where you will find information about fiber and sugars. When considering bread or baked goods, check the amount of **fiber** in the product. It is normal to find one gram or less in products that are made with highly refined flour and other ingredients, but I recommend looking for baked goods with three grams or more, if you are eating them at all. If less than that, you are welcoming that "elephant" we talked about into your body, because that food will quickly turn into sugar.

Also in that section is **Total Sugars** and **Added Sugars**. Most of my clients find the label misleading because sugars noted in grams are hard to equate to a familiar measurement. You have to do a little math (divide by four) to equate it to the teaspoons we normally use to measure. Some foods, such as milk, yogurt, and fruit, contain natural sugars, which is where the "Added Sugars" notation is helpful. It's not unusual to see plain yogurt with six grams of sugar on the nutrition label—that's the milk's natural sugar—but when you see much higher Total Sugars, you know that other ingredients have been added. It's the added sugars that should be avoided, as well as products made from flours that will become sugar after being eaten.

That's where a shift to looking at the actual ingredients is key. Manufacturers list the most prominent ingredient first, followed by others in order of their content. It is important to read through the full list, especially where sugar is concerned. A common practice is to use a variety of added sugars in a product to enhance its flavor and allow the manufacturer to disguise just how much is used.

There are so many different forms of sugar and sweeteners used in food production. The most prominent terms to scan for in that ingredient list would be syrup, sugar and anything ending in "ose", such as dextrose, sucrose and fructose. In addition to these, you may also see:

- Agave nectar
- Fruit juice
- Muscovado
- Barley malt
- Fruit concentrate
- Panocha
- Cane juice

- Honey
- Sweet sorghum
- Corn sweetener
- Maltodextrin
- Treacle
- Dextrin
- Maltol

You may be surprised that I included agave nectar in this list. Had you heard that it was a healthier sweetener? Sadly, agave has more fructose in it than high fructose corn syrup and consuming it regularly can stress your liver.

This was actually a short list of the more common sweeteners. I have seen lists of sixty-one different sweeteners[18], and that didn't include the artificial sweeteners that are so common. I mentioned them back in Chapter 7. They include:

- Aspartame
- Acesulfame K
- Saccharin
- Sucralose
- Acesulfame Potassium
- Neotame

I don't recommend consuming these in your food or beverages because they have negative effects on your body. If you need to sweeten your foods, I suggest you use local raw honey or maple syrup. These are less processed and also offer the benefit of some nutrients but use them sparingly.

One of my clients was in the habit of working out at the gym and had started drinking Gatorade regularly. After all, it is what athletes drink, right? As we worked on adjusting her food and drink selections based on her health goals, I encouraged her to keep a journal of everything she consumed. Gatorade was listed several times on her journal, so I asked her to bring a bottle to our session. When we sat down together, she pulled out the Gatorade bottle and I produced an empty Coke bottle for her to compare. She turned both bottles around and her eyes grew big as they bounced back and forth from one label to the other. They both had a similar amount of sugar. In fact, three of the four ingredients in Gatorade were sugars. No joke! She already knew that she didn't want the chemicals in the sugar free version, so I suggested an alternative: a plain glass of water with the juice of half a lemon, plus a pinch of Himalayan pink salt. It wouldn't have the fancy flavor, but it would provide the electrolyte boost, which is the reason we usually drink a sports drink anyways.

There are other options for sweetening beverages. As I mentioned before, I've begun using Glycine powder as a sweetener. It is a natural amino acid that your body can use, and it has a gentle sweetness that works very well in a cup of coffee or tea. If you want your homemade sports drink or any beverage to taste a bit sweeter, I suggest adding ¼ teaspoon of Glycine to it.

Stevia is a relatively newer sweetener that comes from a plant in the chrysanthemum family. I have grown it in my garden and the leaves do taste sweet when you chew them. Some of my clients have commented that stevia has an aftertaste, but I have found that it is usually because they are using too much. Available in liquid or powder form, I recommend you start with just a few drops of liquid or half a packet of the powder and add more if needed. When choosing stevia in the store, check the ingredient label. When buying packets of powdered stevia, you should look for a brand that has two ingredients: stevia extract and inulin or another fiber source. Many brands have dextrose (recognize that from the list above?) and other ingredients that aren't necessary. A liquid stevia will usually have more than two ingredients.

While we want to believe that everything in the grocery store is beneficial, it is sadly not the truth. Food manufacturers are in business to make a profit and to do that they catch your attention—even prime an addiction—with sweet and salty flavors. For the sake of reclaiming your health, you must be aware of what is in your food and choose foods with ingredients for life.

Put into Action

Explore your refrigerator and pantry, reading the labels and checking ingredients against the lists I've provided. Decide whether each of those foods would support your body or work against it. Is it worth it to continue to eat those that work against you?

Maintaining or Gaining
Weight Healthfully

MANY PEOPLE IN TREATMENT FOR CANCER HAVE REPORTED TO me that their doctor was pressing them to keep their weight up. Their doctor encouraged them to eat whatever they wanted that was high in calories. They suggested milkshakes, donuts, ice cream, pudding—anything that appealed to the patient.

Sadly, there is a common misconception—even among doctors—that simply eating lots of foods that are high in calories will accomplish the goal. However, so many of these foods offer no nutritional value and work against you.

What is the common denominator in these foods? Sugar. While sugar will help you gain weight, it won't be healthy weight. It will be fat, which actually stresses your body more with higher cholesterol, high blood pressure, mood swings and insulin resistance. And we've already talked about the effect sugar has on cancer cells.

Increasing calories is the primary means for gaining weight, so let's find a way to add beneficial calories to your diet. There is a significant difference between high-calorie processed or junk foods, such as a milkshake, and nutrient-dense foods that have higher calories, like an avocado—besides the taste, of course.

Processed foods usually have multiple forms of sweeteners along with grain-based flours—all of which turn to sugar in your body. They also include a variety of chemicals as flavor enhancers and preservatives, which stress your already-challenged digestive and immune systems as they seek to sort, remove or store them.

The body needs food to supply the important macronutrients of fat, protein and carbohydrates. Some good options for foods in these categories to aid in healthy weight gain are:

Healthy fats

Healthy fats fall in three categories:

- Omega-9 fatty acids from avocado, olive oil, almonds and macadamia nuts;
- Short-chain fatty acids from grass-fed butter (such as Kerrygold® brand) and coconut oil; and
- Omega-3 fatty acids from wild-caught fish, cage free egg yolks, walnuts, chia seeds and flaxseeds.

Clean protein

Consuming protein provides valuable nutrients for building muscle and tissue in your body. Given the stress your body is already under, it is important to consider the source of your protein. Did that animal you are eating eat a diet that is natural for its species? So much of our meat supply is farmed in a way that saves costs and increases volume (like cows and fish eating corn), yet does so at the expense of nutritional value. I recommend getting your protein from grass-fed beef, wild-caught cold-water fish (salmon, haddock, cod), organic poultry and cage free whole eggs (the kind that have dark, almost orange yolks). Protein powders are available from many sources, but again, what was the source of the protein from which the powder was made? There are protein powders made from bone broth that can satisfy your need for protein as well as provide the benefits of bone broth I shared earlier. For those who follow a vegetarian or vegan approach, there are protein powders made from ground seeds that can fit your needs. If you are in the habit of eating tofu for protein, I recommend that you look for organic to avoid the high percentage of soy that is raised with excessive pesticides.

Carbohydrates

Most people think of flour-based foods when they hear the term "carbs" or "carbohydrates," so it may surprise you to learn that vegetables and fruit also fall into this category of macronutrients. The key is selecting those vegetables that provide the most benefit. In chapter 5 I shared the importance of eating a variety of colors that represent nutrients, and vegetables also provide valuable fiber and complex carbohydrates your body can use for energy. Root vegetables—yams, parsnips, beets, rutabaga, carrots, and potatoes—can be a valuable source of these in a variety of colors.

While I would suggest that you focus on vegetables, if you feel that you need to add more bulk to your meals, you could include complex carbohydrate sources (those not ground to flour) such as rolled or steel cut oats, quinoa, or brown rice.

Additional tips for gaining or maintaining weight would be:

- **Adding healthy snacks** between meals will increase your daily calorie count and provide the protein and nutrients your body needs to stay energized and maintain or add some weight. These snacks could include a handful of trail mix with little or no dried fruit or chocolate, veggies and hummus, a hard-boiled egg, or live-culture plain Greek yogurt with seeds, nuts, and berries. Choosing a piece of fruit has been shown to reduce anxiety and emotional distress, and pairing that fruit with a nut butter, such as almond butter, helps improve cognitive function and energy levels.

- **Eating five smaller meals throughout the day**. This will be gentler on your digestive system and help you avoid feeling bloated and lethargic after a bigger meal. Though it may seem like you are always eating at first, your body will become accustomed, and you can choose to incorporate protein shakes or smoothies with mostly veggies and some protein for one of those meals. Liquids are more easily digested and, as I've mentioned before, can be an easy way to add calories—so I recommend choosing the ingredients carefully.
- Lest you think that you should not **exercise in order to gain weight**, I would suggest that a better way to gain weight would be to build muscle. I'm not referring to body building, but simply using some weight resistance (which could be your own body weight), yoga and walking to maintain or develop muscles. It may be a challenge to get started if this hasn't been your habit, but I am quite confident you will feel better as you move frequently.

Bottom line, the healthiest way to gain weight is to build muscle, which requires physical activity at least five times a week, as well as nutritious calories to fuel and provide building blocks for the muscle. We will talk more in a later chapter about the benefits of movement (lest you consider "exercise" to be a negative word) as your body navigates this journey.

Put into Action

If you are being encouraged by your medical team to gain weight, do you see the benefit of shifting your strategy to a more healthful approach? What do you see as the first change you need to make in order to maximize nutrient value for your body? Talk about this with your caregiver or a companion. Explaining it to them will help to clarify its importance for you and you will have support as you make the change.

Working Behind the Lines

NOT EVERY BATTLE NEEDS TO BE FOUGHT ON THE FRONT LINES. Military historians will tell you that many battles were effectively won from behind the lines. One example was the battle for Stalingrad in August 1942. Hitler had amassed the largest force in history against a Russian army that was exhausted and poorly equipped. The Russians held on for months, but their leader realized they were no match for Hitler's forces in a frontal assault. Instead, he sent his troops behind enemy lines to attack those who were supporting the Nazi forces. Not prepared to defend themselves, the Nazi's supplies were cut off. Without resources, the Nazi force had to retreat and the German invasion of Russia was effectively repelled. Just as supply is vital for military forces to carry out their mission, so is supply needed for a tumor to grow in your body.

While you may have thought that your battle with cancer was fully dependent on the medical treatment, I'm hoping that you are beginning to see that you have more control than you thought! Too often I speak with cancer patients who adopt their doctors' opinion that food doesn't matter, and they rely on the cancer treatments to do the whole job. Yet, you can make daily choices that will nourish your whole body *and* disrupt the tumors' supply line, just as the Russians did at Stalingrad. Your efforts toward nourishment and disruption can give you a significant advantage in your battle. There are several resources provided by nature that can do this in your body. Here are some of the key players I have found.

Mushrooms

Mushrooms can be found in many different forms around the world. The more common varieties are readily available in grocery stores, while others can be gathered in the wild, and some are best sourced directly from specialty farmers. Given that there are poisonous mushrooms, I would recommend that you *not* try to collect yours in the wild unless you are working with an experienced forager.

Though many consider mushrooms to be a source of fiber and flavor for their food, they also provide antioxidant and antitumor benefits. A vegetarian source of protein, mushrooms also provide vitamins, minerals, trace elements and fiber. The vital microbiome in your digestive system considers these fungi to be a valuable food source for them to thrive, too.

Related to fighting cancer behind the scenes, mushrooms contain antigen-binding lectins that seek out and stick to cancerous and abnormal cells. These lectins effectively label these cells for destruction by your immune system.

Your doctor may have spoken to you about angiogenesis—the growth of new blood vessel networks—which is essential for survival and growth of tumors. Mushrooms have been shown to contain high levels of angiogenesis inhibitors that hinder the development of that support network.[19, 20] Preventing the grown of blood vessels for the tumor is another benefit of targeting behind the lines.

When mushrooms were tested for their antioxidant benefit, the lowly white button mushroom was found to have the strongest levels, followed by the portobello and cremini varieties. Other varieties—reishi, shiitake, maitake, Lion's Mane, and oyster—are often referred to as medicinal mushrooms because of the many cultures that have used them for centuries to support healing. Exploring a variety of these can provide your body with a range of nutrient building blocks to help you fight behind the lines.

How would you prepare these to eat them? You could grill or bake a portobello mushroom like a burger, add mushrooms to a soup or chili, top your salad with some chopped mushrooms, or sauté mushrooms and onions as a side dish. Interestingly, you can further boost the nutritional value of the mushrooms by putting them out in the sun, upside down (gills facing up) for several hours before cooking them.

And if you aren't keen on eating them, there are many reputable sources of mushroom tinctures or capsule forms you may consider.

Astragalus

Astragalus root is a powerful immune-building plant. This is an adaptogen herb that helps the body respond to stress, anxiety and fatigue by helping the body return to balance. Astragalus is a member of the legume family that has been used in traditional Chinese medicine for centuries. The root of four-year-old plants from two species of Astragalus are harvested for use in conjunction with conventional treatments.

Studies have shown that Astragalus has helped patients receiving chemotherapy to recover from its side effects more quickly. In cases of severe chemotherapy symptoms—nausea, vomiting and diarrhea—astragalus has been given intravenously. Not only can this beneficial adaptogen help to reduce symptoms, it has also been shown to increase the effectiveness of chemotherapy.

Recent screenings have shown that components of astragalus—saponins, flavonoids and polysaccharides—provide antioxidant benefit, are able to decrease tumor size and show promise in reversing multidrug resistance.[21]

How do you incorporate astragalus in your diet? There are a

variety of forms that you can find in a health food store, including tincture (liquid extract), capsules, dried herb to make tea, or topical creams. You may benefit from choosing a couple forms—perhaps tincture and topical cream, or capsules (250-500mg of standardized extract up to three times a day) and astragalus tea to drink several times a day—to bring the benefits of astragalus in through multiple routes.

Green Tea

Plants that grow in particularly challenging environments offer components that benefit our bodies. Green tea is one of those plants and its epigallocatechin gallate (EGCG)[22,23] is one of the most powerful nutritional molecules that fights angiogenesis, the formation of new blood vessels for cancer cells.

All tea is made from parts of the Camellia Sinensis plant. Black tea is made from the fermented leaves, but that fermentation process destroys the valuable EGCG, so it is important for you to drink green tea. Japanese green tea, such as Matcha or Sencha, is even richer in EGCG than common Chinese green tea.

Green tea must be steeped for ten minutes to release its catechins, which are effective antioxidants. Once it is steeped, drink it within an hour as it loses the beneficial catechins over time. Drinking two-to-three cups a day will provide sufficient levels in the blood to be spread by capillaries to each cell. When EGCG settles on the surface of cells it blocks the signal that allows the penetration of neighboring tissue by cancer cells and hinders angiogenesis to support the tumor.

You may think that buying a case of bottled green tea would be an easier way to get the benefits of EGCG. I do not recommend that approach because bottled green tea does not have active catechins, and it also has added sweeteners. You won't get the desired benefits unless you brew your own tea.

Be aware that there is caffeine in green tea. If your body is sensitive to caffeine, it would be best to drink the tea earlier in the day.

Curcumin

The growth and spread of cancer cells rely to a large extent on a proinflammatory factor secreted by the cells with the fancy name of NF-kappa B. It is something of a black knight that inhibits apoptosis (cell death) and supports metastases (tumor cell spread). Bharat Aggarwal, Ph.D., from M.D. Anderson Cancer Center, has written that controlling the harmful effects of NF-kappa B in cancer is "a question of life or death." Thankfully, nature has provided us with a substance to help in this effort.

Many cultures in Asia have included turmeric in their daily foods for centuries. Now the world is catching on to its many benefits, including its anti-inflammatory and antioxidant activity. While adding turmeric as a dietary ingredient does not provide the level needed for therapeutic benefit, isolated supplements of curcumin, the key component in turmeric, are now available.

In the case of cancer, high doses of curcumin (four-to-eight grams daily) have been found to be most beneficial and studies continue to explore the mechanisms by which curcumin works.[24] Phytosome curcumin, available online or from specialty stores, is found to have greater absorption because its lecithin formulation causes it to bypass stomach acid to be absorbed in the small intestine where fats are digested and absorbed. The recommendation is to begin with 1,000mg (one gram) twice a day for several days and then work up to multiple grams (four-to-eight grams) daily. I recommend you share the studies referenced in the endnotes with your doctor and discuss the benefits before you incorporate curcumin to support your battle.

Nature provides us with valuable "chemicals" that can support your body in fighting against cells that have gone rogue. These are examples of food as medicine. Incorporate one or a combination of these—one cup of medicinal mushrooms, three cups of home-brewed

green tea, or phytosome curcumin (with your doctor's agreement)—
into your diet regularly to support your body by cutting off the supply
lines for the tumors.

Put into Action

You have read of several forms of support that you can incorporate to
boost your body's ability to take a stand against the cancer cells.
Which one will you explore first? I daresay that at least one of these
has caught your attention. Start there.

Move Your Lymph

MOST EVERYONE IS FAMILIAR WITH THE CARDIOVASCULAR system that helps to pump blood to the body's tissues through its series of arteries, capillaries, and veins. Did you know there is another series of vessels that carry a clear liquid called lymph?

While nutrients and oxygen are delivered to the body through blood, lymph has the task of collecting waste, toxins, and debris while also distributing immune cells through the body. Your lymphatic system is a network of vessels and lymph nodes working together to carry fluids from your tissues to your blood. It is basically your body's inner drainage system. Just as we see in our own neighborhoods, garbage collection is just as important as delivery of mail, water, and other services. Keeping your lymph flowing smoothly is critical for your body's wellbeing.

This system also plays a part in immune function as your lymph nodes receive fluid from the vessels. When bacteria or foreign matter is detected in the lymph, they are trapped, and white blood cells are created to handle the infection. This may cause the lymph node to swell.

The lymph system also helps to keep body fluids in balance so that gravity doesn't cause collection of fluid in lower extremities. When you notice swelling or fluid build-up, it may be in response to injury, or it may be a sign that your lymph system is congested.

If you've ever experienced a garbage strike in your city, you remember the effect of excess garbage piling up. That can happen in your body as well with lymph congestion.

What contributes to this type of congestion? Chronic stress, chronic inflammation, digestive imbalance, and dehydration.

Chronic Stress

Chronic stress contributes to many health issues. One downstream aspect of stress is creation of stress-fighting hormones, which result in free radical waste—the garbage created by various processes in the body—that must be collected by the lymph system and can build up in the lymph nodes.

Chronic Inflammation

Chronic Inflammation causes production of more white blood cells to fight the microbes. These new blood cells, along with the debris that is collected by the lymph, can congest the lymph nodes, and prevent proper flow of lymph through the body.

Digestive Imbalance

The majority of your lymph system surrounds your gut where bacteria and toxins are more likely to enter the body. Digestive imbalance or damaged intestinal villi will have a negative influence on lymph flow and detoxification.

Dehydration

What flows better, a thin fluid or a thick one? I think you would agree that a thin fluid would flow better and the best way to thin the lymph fluid is by drinking water. Dehydration, along with a sedentary life-style, will slow the flow significantly. Unlike the cardiovascular system, the lymph system does not have a pump. It relies on muscle movement and breathing to propel its fluids throughout the body.

Cancer treatment can contribute to lymph congestion by increasing free radical waste, so I want to share some ideas of how you can get things moving better.

Deep Breathing

Deep breathing is a great place to start as it can reduce stress, move the rib cage for better lymph movement and increase the oxygen supply for your body. Our tendency is to breath in a shallow manner most of the time, so you have to focus to really breathe deeply. Start by breathing in through your nose, hold it to the count of 5, then exhale slowly through your mouth. Repeat this two-to-three times each session. I recommend doing this at least three times a day.

Drinking Plenty of Water

Lymph contains 95% water, so drinking plenty of water is vital for healthy lymph function. In fact, your body relies on a steady water supply for all organs to function properly. We lose water from our bodies through breathing, talking, sweating, and peeing, so it is impor-tant to replenish what is lost. Adding a squeeze of lemon or lime can speed the hydration process, encourage an alkaline environment in your body and boost lymph flow.

Though I recommend starting with half your body weight in ounces of water each day, simply drinking more water is a first step. If your practice has been to drink flavored liquids, would you be willing to trade out one of those for water? Once that first trade is working for you, consider swapping another flavored drink for water. One swap at a time can move you more comfortably to drinking mostly water, and your body will benefit.

Regular Exercise or Movement

Regular exercise or movement has many benefits, including helping to move lymph through your body and clearing congestion. It's one of the easiest ways to improve your lymph flow. Walking is perhaps the simplest form of movement for most people, but what I have found is the key to regular movement is finding a form that you enjoy. You may prefer swimming or dancing or playing with your dog. Activity that moves your arms, legs and torso helps to move your lymph while also stimulating blood circulation and oxygen supply to your cells and reducing toxin buildup. If you are currently spending a lot of time in bed, you could support lymph flow by having someone pump your legs as though you were riding a bike, and bend and lift your arms. Laying with your legs and arms extended toward the ceiling allows gravity to support lymph movement. Many people find laying on the floor with their buttocks against the baseboard and their legs up the wall to be relaxing, and it helps move their lymph.

Dry Skin Brushing

Dry skin brushing is a technique from Ayurvedic traditions that can boost circulation, lymphatic flow and detoxification. A dry brush is often designed to fit the palm of your hand and is made of soft, natural bristles. Beginning at your feet, brush up the front, sides and back of your legs with gentle strokes, always moving toward your heart. Then brush your arms starting at your wrists and moving toward your heart. Brush your belly in a clockwise motion that will also help to improve your natural digestive flow. The best time to dry brush is before you take a shower or bathe, as dry brushing will also help to exfoliate dead skin cells that can be washed away.

Massage

Having a massage is another way to improve both the flow of blood and of lymph. Lymphatic drainage massage is a specialized massage designed to reduce congestion, help your cells release toxic buildup, and flush excess fluid. Massage is relaxing and can also reduce pain. If you have not had a massage before, tell the masseuse what your concerns are and whether there are areas of your body that need to be avoided. You may find that this will be a valuable addition to your care.

As a patient in treatment for cancer, I'm sure that you have heard your doctor talk about the lymph nodes and checking them for the spread of cancer cells is a regular practice. If you didn't know why this was important before, perhaps you have a better understanding now.[25] Those who find their body seems to be retaining fluids, may find these methods of moving lymph will help reduce swelling or puffiness.[26] Choosing at least one or two of these ways to support the flow of lymph through your body will help you weather the challenges of treatment more comfortably.

Put into Action

I hope you have begun to drink more water based on Chapter 7. Now choose one of the activities—movement, dry brushing, or massage—to begin to get your lymph moving.

Sleep is Non-negotiable

It may seem surprising for sleep to be covered in a book about nutrients and food, yet sleep is key to many aspects of physical and mental health. Studies link sleep deprivation with a host of diseases and symptoms ranging from obesity and diabetes, to depression and anxiety. Sleep is key to keeping the immune system strong as it is the time when the body gets a break from the demands of the day and can recharge and renew. If you are choosing foods that provide a wide range of beneficial nutrients, but not sleeping, your body will still struggle.

Many cleanup functions happen while we sleep—memories are stored, hormones are restocked, toxins are processed, tissue is repaired, and immune cells are produced.[27]

Sadly, it is reported that seventy million Americans have trouble sleeping. Are you one of them?

Sleep troubles come in many varieties. Do you have trouble shutting down your thoughts, or actually falling asleep? Perhaps you used to have trouble sleeping until you began cancer treatments and now your body is demanding more sleep.

Do you fall asleep easily but wake often during the night? Does your significant other snore, or do they complain that you do? If you find it hard to drag yourself out of bed in the morning, you are likely not sleeping well, and it is both decreasing your brain function and affecting your body's ability to heal.

Do you ascribe to the belief that sleep is overrated? If so, you may not realize that skimping on sleep can decrease the blood flow to your brain, which disrupts thinking, memory and concentration. And if you combine unsupported sleep apnea with fewer hours allowed for sleep, you are seriously limiting the oxygen that is reaching your brain and your cells.

Scientists have discovered fascinating new research that the brain has a special "waste management system" that works while you sleep to get rid of toxins, including the brain plaque that is thought to contribute to age-related memory issues. Without healthy sleep, this cleaning crew doesn't have enough time to do their job and trash collects, causing brain fog and memory problems. Quality sleep is essential to wellness![28]

My client, Kristen, came to me for help to improve her immune system and energy levels. She was surprised when I not only suggested shifting the foods she was eating, but also focused on her sleep. After only a couple coaching sessions she was commenting that she was amazed at the difference a good night's sleep had made in how she felt and functioned during the day. In her words, "getting a good night's sleep consistently can change everything." Keep reading and I will share the tips that helped Kristen.

Block the Blue at Night

Sleep is ultimately the gift of your pineal gland. Following your circadian rhythm, this ant-sized lobe in your brain secretes melatonin, a neurotransmitter and hormone of which you may have heard. Melatonin suppresses the activity of other neurotransmitters and helps calm the brain to prepare for sleep. But there's a catch...

The pineal gland secretes melatonin largely in response to darkness. Thanks to Edison's light bulb and a myriad of technological advances, we rarely experience much darkness after the sun goes down. Your evening activity choices can get in the way of natural sleep-supporting chemical shifts by confusing your brain about whether or not it is night.[29]

Electronic devices emit blue light which makes your brain think it is daytime when it isn't. Using these devices at night disrupts your circadian rhythm and impairs the secretion of melatonin. Many devices have the capability to filter the blue light at sundown, but they need to be set to do so. If your computer doesn't have a nighttime setting, you can download the F.LUX app to help with this. If you watch TV at night, you can wear blue light blocking glasses to protect yourself from this disruption.

If your sleep pattern has been disrupted, you can begin to reset your circadian rhythm by getting direct sunshine into your eyes soon after waking. Granted, bad weather outside can seem like a hindrance, but if you can put a robe or coat on and sit outside for five-to-ten minutes right after waking up, you will begin to experience a shift. Should being outside not be an option for you, get right by a window without curtains and look outside for five-to-ten minutes to get the light in your eyes.

Avoid Stimulation in the Evening

Activity that stimulates your body will usually raise your cortisol levels and hinder the release of melatonin. This could include listening to loud music or watching violent movies or even the evening news. Regular exercise can help to counter insomnia, yet vigorous exercise in the evening may energize you and keep you awake. Consider an evening stretching class or calming yoga to set the stage for sleep.

If you have ever tried to go to bed when worried or angry, you know how that hinders sleep. Try to settle any emotional troubles before bedtime with a positive message to the other person, or journaling three-to-five things for which you are thankful. There's a reason the Bible encourages us not to let the sun go down on our anger. Gratitude and forgiveness benefit you and also support better sleep!

Quiet Your Digestion

This particularly powerful tip surprises many. If you struggle with insomnia or light, restless sleep, it is recommended that you not eat for a full three hours before bed. This allows your body to focus its energy on restorative activities rather than digestion once you are in bed.

The exception to this is in cases of hypoglycemia. If you experience episodes of low blood sugar, it is good to have a small protein-rich snack before bed.

Many people reach for a glass of wine or alcohol to relax before bed, yet this can actually cause you to wake in the middle of the night.[30] Some of the cancer patients I spoke to reported that they discovered that alcohol wasn't their friend during treatment for this reason. Processing that beverage requires your liver to stop what it would normally do so that it can attend to the alcohol which can hinder its normal nighttime processes. As a soothing alternative, try a cup of hot tea or bone broth, or a mixture of warm almond or coconut milk, a teaspoon of vanilla and a few drops of stevia. This tasty beverage may increase serotonin in your brain to help you sleep.

You are probably already aware of how your body handles caffeine. Its metabolism is highly individual. Genetically, some people are slow metabolizers and find that caffeine affects them for a longer period of time after consumption. If you have noticed that you are sensitive to caffeine, be aware that sodas, tea, energy drinks, and chocolate also have caffeine. It would be better to avoid these from mid-afternoon to bedtime and instead choose herbal chamomile tea in the evening.

Create an Ideal Sleep Environment

A cooler temperature is more conducive to sleep, so turn the temperature down in your bedroom (if not your whole house) at night. If you find yourself still getting hot when you sleep, try bamboo sheets. The fabric is recognized for regulating temperature exchange and keeping the sleeper cool. They are also moisture-wicking and hypoallergenic.

Make sure the room is dark. If you have a streetlight shining outside your bedroom window, try a light-blocking shade to make the room dark and help to balance your circadian rhythm. Check sources of light in your bedroom. Does your alarm clock have a bright light? It may be playing a part in your sleep challenges. Even a TV in your bedroom can be a hindrance—watching it just before going to sleep, or having it on after you fall asleep, will disrupt your circadian rhythm and keep you from sleeping deeply.

If you tend to keep your phone or other devices by your bed at night, put them on "airplane" mode and turn off the location services. Ideally, put your WIFI router on a timer so it shuts off while you are sleeping. This will give your body a break from the EMF radiation that these emit in your home.

Explore whether you like having sound while you sleep or prefer silence. If your sleeping partner snores, ear plugs can rescue your relationship. Some find total silence a bit disconcerting and benefit from sound therapy to induce a peaceful mood and lull them to sleep. Soothing nature sounds, wind chimes, a fan or binaural beat music can help with sleep. With a little experimentation, you can find what's right for you.

Create a Bedtime Transition Routine

When you are reprogramming your circadian rhythm, it is important to go to bed at a consistent time. Setting a routine can help to train your body that's it's time to go to bed. Your routine may begin about an hour before bedtime and include some of the following:

- Turning off electronics
- Listening to calming music or a guided meditation
- Taking a bath with Epsom salts added to the water
- Reading a calming book (if on an electronic reader, set for black background)
- Writing in a journal
- Playing or snuggling with a pet
- Washing your face and brushing your teeth

You can be thankful if you are able to sleep seven-to-nine hours each night without difficulty. Yet, if you are one of the many people who struggle with sleep, I encourage you to make it a priority and explore a combination of these tips for several nights each. Treat this like an experiment, recognizing that your sleep will not be fixed right away. Give it time and keep exploring different combinations of these tips. Sleep is vital for healing, and that's a priority for you at this time in your life.

Put into Action

If you experience sleep challenges, what have I shared that piqued your interest? That may be the best place to begin. As with any experimental process, it would be good to keep notes of what you change and how your body responds.

Your Body in Motion

We tend to think that food is all that nourishes our body, but there is more. In addition to "sustaining with food or nutriment," nourish also means to "supply with what is necessary for life, health and growth." Movement falls into that aspect of nourishment for your body.

Prior to your diagnosis, were you physically active? Did you walk regularly, or participate in a dance or exercise class? Perhaps you enjoyed lifting weights at the gym, or you preferred the calm breathing and stretching of a yoga class.

What do you remember enjoying about your exercise? Being outside in nature? The demands, and aches, when you sought to push to a new level? Even when you pushed hard, did you feel better afterward—even refreshed?

Or did you view exercise as torture, and you avoided it at all costs? I don't ask to make you feel guilty, but like the rest of this book, to help you going forward.

What has been your practice since your diagnosis and the start of your treatment? Have you found yourself sleeping more, or staying sedentary far more than in the past?

If fatigue, depression, and general malaise have been your experience with treatment, I would encourage you to get your body in motion.

What's your first response to that statement? Shock? Disbelief? A sarcastic comment? That's okay. All I ask is that you hear what I am trying to convey.

Your body is designed to move. When you sit or lay for long periods of time, your joints become stiff and your muscles can actually weaken and shrink. Did you know that many doctors now believe that sitting for extended periods of time produces similar effects in the body as long-term smoking?[31] That's not a good thing.

I have had many clients whose jobs entailed long hours at a desk. They bemoaned feeling tethered—or maybe even chained—in that place and the limits it presented. Yet there are some creative ways you can insert movement. Many are requesting that their employers provide a standing desk converter—a platform that sits on top of the desk and can be used at the lowest setting when sitting or adjusted to higher positions for standing. Another option, depending on the setting of your office and whether you always talk on a phone with a cord that limits your movement, is to get in the habit of walking around while you are talking on the phone. Even setting an alarm to remind you to get up and walk for a few minutes each hour or so, can provide benefits to your body and actually refresh your brain.

There are many benefits to movement. Remember what was shared earlier about the lymphatic system being important for collecting and removing trash from the body, in addition to transporting immune cells. Unlike the cardiovascular system, which is pumped by the heart, the lymphatic system does not have a pump. It relies on muscle movement to "pump" it around.

Your movement isn't limited to when you are upright. If you are needing bedrest, your body can get similar benefit from moving your arms and legs. Arms can be raised over your head and moved around in circles, bending and straightening at the elbow, while legs can be raised up toward the ceiling while straight and then bent at the knee to press toward your chest. Whether you move on your own or have the help of someone, this movement not only pumps the lymph through your body but also lubricates your joints.

Good news! You don't need to go back to the gym—unless that is a motivating place for you. Something as simple as walking can be invigorating and therapeutic. One of the ladies that I interviewed said that she was walking several miles outside every day. She would bundle up if it was cold and have covering if it rained. She reported that she felt rejuvenated after walking outside—escaping her all-too-familiar apartment to see the outdoor beauty around her, smelling the change in the air with different weather patterns, feeling the air in her lungs as it brought life with each inhale, hearing sounds of nature intertwined with the city. All of these were a highlight of her day. They lifted her mood, drew in oxygen for her cells and even helped her sleep better at night.

Following these simple guidelines can help to ease the transition toward a new way to nourish and support your body. Introducing movement back into your routine is a way to support your body for better function through your treatment and beyond. Ideally, it will become a habit for the rest of your life—it's that important.

Begin Slowly and Gently

There is no magic distance, time, or speed for everyone. Perhaps you start with a walk around your block, or just park further away from your office or the store so you walk through the parking lot. Even a bathroom break can provide an opportunity to move and you can make the most of it by going to the bathroom located the farthest from your current location. As mentioned above, there are added benefits if the place you walk also engages your senses.

Find a Buddy

You may share my tendency to let other demands in your life super-sede your own needs. How long is your task list? What is the weather like outside? Maybe your energy feels low and you doubt that you can make it out there and back. Having a buddy and a scheduled time to rendezvous always helps me fulfill my exercise plans. After all, it's far more fun to have someone with whom you can talk and share the activity. If you find yourself walking alone, you could consider listening to music, audio books or podcasts to keep you company.

Choose an Activity You Enjoy

You certainly won't persist if you don't enjoy yourself. Walking may be a starting place, but you can also explore bicycling, yoga, Pilates, strength training, or one of the many forms of dancing. If you were a runner before your diagnosis, you may be able to continue at a gentler pace or shorter distance. The American College of Sports Medicine now has a certification for Cancer Exercise Trainers, so you could inquire in your area if you feel that having a trainer would be of bene-fit. Listen to your body. I believe it will tell you what is beneficial, and more times than not, my experience has been that even when I didn't feel up to the movement, when I finished I felt much better.

Focus on Consistency

Just as you protect time on your calendar for your medical appoint-ments, set times for movement in your calendar. You may start with just three times a week but work up to moving daily—and the normal movement around your house doesn't count, assuming you don't walk laps around your house for an extended period. Change up the types of movement, if that would keep it more interesting for you.

Try Grounding

Have you heard of grounding, or earthing? It refers to the simple practice of being barefoot outdoors in order to connect with the Earth's electrons. If you have ever walked barefoot on the beach and felt energized and restored, you have experienced grounding.

Our modern practice of wearing shoes with rubber or plastic soles has separated us from the flow of the Earth's electrons. Yet one of the simplest health interventions is available right beneath our feet.

There are many scientific studies[32] that have demonstrated the benefits of grounding, but the most effective will be for you to explore it yourself. Kick off your shoes and go outside. Spend time sitting, standing or walking with your feet on grass, soil, sand, or even concrete. These are all conductive surfaces that will allow your body to absorb electrons from the Earth. Do this consistently for a week and note what you notice about your sleep, your level of pain,[33] your level of stress,[34] and your overall mood.

Beyond actual time spent barefoot outside, there are many resources available to enhance grounding in your home. These include mattress covers, chair pads, floor pads and chairs that can be grounded. Old-fashioned leather-soled shoes and sandals also conduct electrical grounding if you are not comfortable being barefoot.

Barbara, a client I worked with a few years ago, struggled with joint pain and anxiety. When she came to me, she was taking over-the-counter painkillers several times a day and had developed digestive distress. I suggested that she switch to using the phytosome curcumin I mentioned in Chapter 11 because the over-the-counter painkillers can damage the gut. Then we began the process of shifting her food choices to remove foods that aggravate joint pain and promote anxiety. I also recommended that she begin to include grounding in her daily routine. Barbara did some limited gardening in her yard and decided to go barefoot while she did this, as well as kick off her shoes and walk barefoot in the grass for at least ten minutes if she wasn't gardening. She also began to sit in a chair with her bare feet on her concrete porch when she read each day. We met again two weeks after she had begun this practice and she declared, "I'm not sure what has helped the most, the change in food or the grounding. I must admit I was skeptical about the grounding, since it usually hurt to move around. I figured I needed to at least try. My gut feels so much better with the change in food, but my whole body feels better with grounding. Who knew it could be this simple?"

There are so many aspects to maintaining the health of our intricate bodies. Movement plays an important role. Walking is a foundational movement from toddlerhood throughout our lives. As unique as each of us are, there are varied forms of movement that incite joy and maintain flexible joints and strong muscles. Find the form of movement that will support both your body and your mind and incorporate grounding in the process. I believe you will discover a refreshed mood and feel more balanced in your body when you do.

Put into Action

What forms of movement did you enjoy before your diagnosis? Is this something that you can resume, or do you feel you need to find a alternate movement to support your body? If you did not have a habit of movement before your diagnosis, I would suggest that you start simply with grounding or walking near your home. Whatever your choice, keep notes of how you feel during and after your movement as you progress through a week.

Your Chemo Tolerance Toolbox

My purpose in writing this book is to equip you with a variety of tools you can adopt for your toolbox to help approach your cancer journey from a place of strength. Your medical team will celebrate your survival at the end of your treatment, yet I seek to also celebrate that you thrived in the process.

Maybe the word *thrive* had never occurred to you in relation to this journey. When you picked up this book were you mostly focused on surviving? If so, I hope that you are now more open to the possibility of thriving!

What do you picture when you read the word *thrive*? Perhaps it's having strength to do your daily activities. Feeling fueled in your body by the food you eat. Sleeping well and waking refreshed. Moving through your day with a positive attitude.

There will likely be days that are harder, when your body feels like it is heavily protesting the treatment you are receiving. You may feel tired. You may even feel weepy and frustrated. Acknowledge when those feelings arise and affirm your belief that you will come through.

What you may need at those times is a little detox, leading up to and following the chemo treatment. The treatment is intended to kill cancer cells, and once that is done, those dead cells need to be removed from the body. The dead cells and any other residual effects of the treatment need to be flushed, which is where detox comes in.

Doesn't the body detox on its own each day? Yes, it does. We are exposed to countless external substances through our food, water and air that must be filtered and removed (detoxed), and there are also substances made in our bodies that need to be removed. Your lymph system and liver play a big part in this process.

When your system cannot keep up with what we are exposed to in normal daily living plus what is added in the course of your cancer treatment, the backup plan is to shunt excess into storage in your fat cells. Your body will slow down, symptoms will become more pronounced and you will feel worse.

But you can help your body with the detox process by adding in some external support using castor oil packs, detox baths and some rebounding. Several people I interviewed recommended doing castor oil packs and a detox bath daily for the week leading up to and following chemo.

Castor Oil Packs

Castor oil is extracted from the seeds of the castor bean and has been used to support improved health for centuries. By using it externally as a pack over the right side and abdomen, the body absorbs it through the skin into lymphatic circulation where it can both soothe and assist in cleansing.

Using a castor oil pack supports relaxation and the parasympathetic nervous function, as well as reducing inflammation and supporting better balance in your gut bacteria.[35]

The pack is most effective when placed over the liver, which is located on the right side of the body below the breast and down to the bottom of the rib cage. It is good to apply the pack and leave it on for at least an hour. It could be applied prior to taking a nap, or while watching TV or a movie. Daily use provides the greatest benefit, but if this is not possible, try for at least four consecutive days per week. Supplies you will need:

- Cold-pressed Castor Oil
- Cotton or wool flannel, 36" x 18" in size
- A garbage bag or saran wrap
- A hot-water bottle or heating pad

Rub a generous amount of castor oil on the skin in the area of the liver, over both the front and back ribs. Place the flannel over the area where you applied the oil, then wrap that in saran wrap or the folded garbage bag to prevent any oil from getting on bedding or furniture. Place the heat source over the plastic and relax.

Making a homemade castor oil pack can be a bit messy. There is a pack that I have used that can be drizzled with castor oil and then actually tied on your body with minimal mess or fuss. You can find the link for this pack on my book portal.

Detox Baths

Epsom Salts is magnesium sulfate in crystal form. Most of us are deficient in magnesium, so being able to absorb it through the skin is beneficial for relieving aches and pains, reducing inflammation, and supporting better digestion. The sulfate helps to flush toxins from your cells to be moved out of the body. The addition of baking soda to the detox bath further enhances the ability to clear toxins from the body. These baths are very relaxing and can provide a simple way to support your body for sleep and recovery.

Your skin is quite porous and laying in hot water prompts your pores to open to allow the minerals in the bath to be absorbed. Adding these minerals creates a reverse osmosis effect where the minerals are drawn in and exchanged with salts that are drawn out of your body along with toxins. Be mindful of not getting the water too hot so that you don't get overheated. Unlike a hot tub, the bath water will be cooling down. Since the toxins are drawn into the water, it is recommended that you stand up as the water drains and turn on the shower for a quick rinse before getting out.

To prepare your detox bath, you need:

- 2 cups of Epsom salts
- 1 cup of baking soda
- 4 drops each of rosemary and juniper berry essential oils (optional)

Add the baking soda under the stream of water to help it dissolve. If you have ever tried to put oil in water you know they don't mix effectively, so hold some of the Epsom salts in your hand and drip the essential oil drops onto the salts. Wait a few seconds for absorption and then dump the Epsom salts into the stream of water as the tub is filling. This will help the essential oils not float on the top where they may be too concentrated and uncomfortable. These essential oils provide a dual benefit—aromatherapy during your bath and added drawing capability.

Filling the tub with enough water to submerge most of your body up to your neck is the best. If you don't have a bathtub, you can do foot soaks with ½ cup of Epsom salts and ¼ cup of baking soda, and one drop each of the essential oils. Rinse your feet when you finish to ensure that toxins don't remain on your skin to be reabsorbed.

Whether you are laying in a bathtub or soaking your feet in a foot bath, try to soak for at least 15-20 minutes, or until the water is cool.

Rebounding

While not as relaxing as the castor oil pack or detox bath, rebounding provides a simple way to move your lymphatic system. The equipment you need is a mini trampoline, unless you happen to have a big one in your back yard. Some mini trampolines provide just the base, while some have a handle to provide stability while you bounce.

Rebounding on a mini trampoline creates an increased gravitational resistance, which opens up your lymphatic valves, encouraging lymph flow. Though considered a low-impact activity, the up and down movement against the force of gravity promotes a surge of lymphatic drainage. This improves your circulation and facilitates beneficial detox.

Start with just two minutes of rebounding your first day to see how your body responds. Your movement can be as simple as lightly bouncing without your feet leaving the pad. Lymphatic flow will still be improved.

As you become more confident on the mini trampoline, you can try higher jumps and longer periods of time in the activity. There are a number of rebounding videos available on YouTube that could even inspire a new form of movement if you really enjoy it.

Don't have a mini trampoline? You could resort to the good ol' jumping jack, provided your feet and legs are up to it. Start with just a few and work your way up.

Hydration

We have already talked about the importance of hydration, and I want to offer a reminder here. A key to helping the body flush toxins out is having plenty of water in your system. Don't forget to drink half your body weight in water each day. If you weigh 160 pounds, that translates to a goal of drinking eighty ounces or more of water daily. You can squeeze lemon juice into your water for flavor and to aid in clearing the liver, but don't float the squeezed lemon wedge in your water after squeezing it. The oils in the skin of a lemon absorb and hold any pesticides used as they were grown—and you don't want those released in your water for you to drink.

I offer these as tools in your toolbox—not required but beneficial. I have regularly recommended detox baths to my clients both for added absorption of magnesium and the benefit of gently removing toxins. Of the clients for whom I recommended castor oil packs, one stands out in my memory. After getting the supplies and talking through the process, Sharon was eager to experience the pack for herself. She was the mom of three small children which was part of her challenge in healing—she put most of her energy into caring for and supervising them, leaving little allocated time for her own care. We had talked about the importance of filling her own cup so that she could pour out for others, and she admitted that it was a struggle to prioritize herself.

The day we discussed the castor oil pack, I presented her with a small gift—a tiara—to symbolize that she was the queen of the home and I encouraged her to teach her children that when she wore the tiara she was not to be disturbed. Sharon beamed with delight, remembering her younger years when she had great fun dressing up and playing with her friends. It took some planning, but she made her tiara time a priority, starting with short periods and slowly extending the time. When we met again, she reported that her children played right along as though it were a game, and she had definitely felt her mood balance out after giving herself the gift of time coupled with the castor oil pack. Whether you have small children or older ones at home, prioritize time for you to relax with the help of the castor oil pack or detox bath. I'm certain that you will notice a difference as Sharon did.

Put into Action

Which of these tools interests you? You may be able to try one of these right away or need a little time to collect supplies. The key is to experiment with them and see how your body responds.

Dissolving Fear

WHAT WERE YOUR FIRST THOUGHTS WHEN YOU RECEIVED YOUR diagnosis? Since memories are generally set when we feel strong emotions, it is likely that you remember that moment well.

Many have reported that there was an immediate rush of fear, followed by disbelief. Some experienced a strange paralysis of mind and body—with their thoughts blurring in a fog and a feeling that they were watching the moment through a smudged window. Did you have a similar experience?

Fear seems to block our life force when we need full access most. It is a natural human response, yet if we dwell there too long it will actually depress our immune system, working against us at a cellular level. Instead, you can choose to nourish your life and appreciate its true value.

It may seem hard—even impossible at times—to shift your thoughts to a more positive focus. I encourage you to be gentle with yourself and practice it in short intervals. If you are a parent, think back to when your child was very young and super inquisitive. She explored her environment in a tactile manner—touching, tasting, manipulating to learn more. If she was drawn to something you did not want her to have, you may have moved her away from that item, saying "no" as you did. Once was not enough, was it? She kept coming back to it, and you either continued to move her away or finally moved the object out of reach and distracted her with something else. You can do something similar with your thoughts—countering the negative ones with a positive reframe or choosing another focus to engage your mind. I have some ideas to share that may be helpful for you.

The very common fear that arises with the initial diagnosis and the related flurry of doctor appointments is the feeling that the world is spinning out of control. You may also have experienced runaway fears, with your imagination trying to fill in unknowns for your future ... usually with worst-case scenarios.

This was what Shawn reported to me when I interviewed her. She was thankful that a friend, Kathy, was with her when her doctor informed her of her cancer diagnosis, because the initial rush of fear completely blurred both her hearing and vision. Though she didn't feel the room spinning as one might with vertigo, she definitely felt as if she were on a carnival ride that had lifted her above the actual scene in the doctor's office. The warmth of Kathy's hand grasping hers brought her back down into her chair and helped her focus once again, but on the drive home her imagination launched into vivid scenes of negative outcomes that raised her heart rate and stirred anxiety.

Kathy wisely asked her to share some of those scenes and, upon their arrival at Shawn's house, encouraged her to breathe deeply and fix her eyes on a beautiful flower in her front garden. Kathy reminded her that she had a home, a family, many friends who would be with her in the journey, and that she could make choices along the way. She didn't need to be swept up in the swift current of oncology and lose her power to make decisions.

That is one of the messages of this book. You need not surrender your will to the doctors, but rather have continued power to choose how you will walk this path. Remember that your doctors have experience with cancer and traditional treatments, but they are focused there, not on supporting the rest of your body. They are also rarely even aware of how your mind and spirit play a part. Many of the cancer survivors I spoke with reported a tremendous sense of urgency, stirred by the doctors and their internal fear, to jump into a treatment plan. They used phrases like "I felt like I was picked up by flood waters" or "it took over everything." Did you feel this way, too? Moving quickly into a treatment plan is understandable, since we naturally want the cancer out of our bodies, and swift action helps us to channel the anxiety we are feeling. Some of my interviewees expressed regret that they had not chosen to take a week or so to review their options and "get their feet back under them."

Have you also wondered what contributed to the cancer, why it developed in you? "Why me?" is a question asked in so many situations. No doubt, you have found that dwelling there keeps you stuck in an emotional mud hole.

Rather than dwelling in that mud hole, try switching the question to: "how can I grow through this journey?" Acknowledge that all these questions and feelings are clear signs that your mind and body are mobilizing in an effort to protect you, to keep you safe in the familiar. Yet clinging to the familiar may limit you on your journey. When you have come to a place where you can release "Why me?" and begin to shift your question, you may find a wide range of possibilities in the opportunity to cultivate a new aspect of life as you grow through this new journey.

You have likely talked to others who are currently in cancer treatment or have come through the journey. The ones who inspire and uplift are likely the ones who have shifted their focus to the second question – "how can I grow through this journey?" Though they didn't start here, they may have even adopted the uncommon perspective of 'this cancer is a gift to help me learn and grow.'

Cynthia Besteman, owner and founder of Violets Are Blue, said, "The darkest period of your life may actually reveal a beautiful gift. Be it family, friends, a new way you want to live your life or even letting go of toxic people and things in your life. Stay open during illness to look for these gifts. They are there."[36]

There are other fears that arise in this journey—this battle—with cancer. Some have a fear of being alone, which is common even among those who are not sick. Loneliness often causes more suffering than physical pain. When we are venturing into the unknown, it is always encouraging to have someone beside us, even if they don't have any more answers than we do.

Another aspect of being alone is not being free to talk about your thoughts—your dreams and your fears—with others. Positive thinking is promoted by many, but Dr. Bernie Spiegel, who conducts support groups for people who are seriously ill, reminds his patients not to let themselves be locked into what he calls "the prison of positive thinking." Voicing your thoughts to someone who is supportive can help you release them, while still returning to focus on the positive outcome. Especially with those who are close to you—spouse, partner, family members or friends—opening the conversation and encouraging them to voice their thoughts to you will remove the barriers that make you feel alone. I provide some suggestions of support groups, both online and in person, in the book portal.

You may also find yourself afraid of being a burden. This is particularly common among those who have themselves been caregivers and are now needing to be the recipient of care from others. Actress Maura Tierney said, "It's a life-changing thing to be in a position of needing help and being so lucky as to get it. You can't just take care of everybody else all the time. That's almost as perspective-changing as the illness."

To spend your life always giving and not willingly receiving can be stifling. Look closely at nature and you will see that there is an ebb and flow, a give and take, and we are part of that. Start by letting those around you know what you need for support. If they are not able to provide it, bless and release them from your request, and ask another. Your fear may be that their inability to support you is a measure of your value, but it may actually be a reflection of their own limiting beliefs.

As you work through your fears, there are some strategies that may help you:

- **Slow down.** Resist the urge to make major decisions quickly. Take a few days to nurture yourself while you research and explore your options, including selecting your medical team. If you doubt that you are ready to fight this battle, you may want to talk with your doctor about delaying the start of treatment while you take a few weeks to prepare physically and mentally. And if you are already in treatment, don't beat yourself up about decisions you made. Give yourself grace and choose tools that will support you.

- **Nourish your body and mind.** Consider healthful lifestyle changes that would support your body. If you have been in the habit of eating fast food and staying up late, explore ways to nourish your body with better food choices and more sleep as I have mentioned in previous chapters. Take walks outside, preferably in a park or woods with lots of trees and plants. I touched on grounding in Chapter 14 and will share more about connecting with nature in the next chapter. Give yourself the gift of grounding—connecting barefoot with grass, sand or dirt as you walk or sit—to realign your electrical energy by connecting with the earth. It is recognized as a simple way to bring calm and reduce pain.

- **Choose whom to tell.** Not everyone in your life will be able to provide the support you need. Some will reflect their own insecurities and fears back to you, which may

undermine your efforts, so be selective initially in the
friends and family members with whom you share.

- **Use the internet wisely.** We have all experienced
  the rabbit hole of research on the web. Hopefully, you
  have realized that not everything you read there is truth,
  and there seems to be a propensity for presenting the
  negative information first. Select your search terms
  carefully and read what you find with a grain of salt so to
  speak. Recognize that Google actively pushes alternative
  medicine information lower in the search results. Also,
  avoid the temptation to do your research late at night
  when the house is quiet. You will be sacrificing valuable
  sleep time and may hinder your ability to get to sleep as
  you contemplate what you have read. If you find that
  research adds stress, you may ask a friend or family
  member to do specific research for you.

Fear is experienced in the mind, and when dwelt on, has a significant effect on the body. Awareness of the fears that arise in your
thoughts is beneficial in that it alerts you to potential concerns. Do
you find fears move through your mind quickly, or are you dwelling
on them? Fueling the fear with rumination will keep you frozen in
place as that fear grows out of proportion. Take a deep breath. You
are human. Acknowledge your fear without judgement and consider
how to respond. Perhaps you need to journal a conversation with
yourself, reminding yourself of all the times you have faced hard
things and come through stronger. Or you may need to voice your
fear to a companion whom you know will be supportive. Fear is part
of being alive, yet it does not get to define our life.

Put into Action

Sit down with a piece of paper and skim through this chapter again.
When you read a question that resonates, write down your response.

No one will read this, so record your raw emotions and thoughts. Then write a response as you would want to be supported—put it in the voice of someone who you feel would stand by you to listen and respond with affirmation and redirection, as Kathy did for Shawn. Lastly, which of the 4 strategies I shared, do you need to implement and why?

Restore Your Body in Nature

When you are feeling the effects of growing stress levels pressing down on you, or a frantic buzzing in your mind, what do you do for relief? We have already talked about facing fear and the stress it brings, and I have mentioned the benefit of being outside. If taking a walk out in nature has been your response, you already experience the benefit of forest bathing or Shinrin-yoku.

This ancient practice of visiting a forest and breathing in its air is used as a natural remedy for mounting stress and mental fatigue. The point is to take a trip into the forest or even a copse of trees to soak in and fully experience your surroundings.

We are increasingly disconnected from the natural world. Urbanization continues to drive development, with estimates that 68% of the world's population will live in urban areas by 2050. These environments, full of steel, glass and concrete, are associated with increased anxiety and cardiovascular health concerns.

Spending time in nature has been a part of many cultures for centuries, and only now are we developing the technology to validate the benefits that our ancestors valued. In Nordic countries, businesses build time into their employees' work schedules to allow them to get outdoors to refresh. Whether they have their lunch in a park or walk in a nearby forest, their employers recognize that allowing this time for outdoor activity (even in their cold, snowy winters) results in better health and performance.

Tim Beatley, Teresa Heinz Professor of Sustainable Communities, in the Department of Urban and Environmental Planning at the University of Virginia, says, "We are hard-wired from evolution to need and want contact with nature. To have a healthy life, emotionally and physically, requires this contact. The empirical evidence of this is overwhelming: exposure to nature lowers our blood pressure, lowers stress and alters mood in positive ways, enhances cognitive functioning, and in many ways makes us happy. Exposure to nature is one of the key foundations of a meaningful life."[37]

Indeed, scientists have studied the benefits and discovered that forest bathing:

- Increases immune function
- Reduces cortisol and increases parasympathetic nervous system activity
- Decreases scores for anger, depression, fatigue and confusion
- Improves heart rate variability and blood pressure levels

Any natural setting works, particularly wooded areas with conifer trees such as cypress, pine, cedar or juniper. It need not be a large area, but one where you can walk at a comfortable pace, explore the plants, sit in quiet meditation, or even lie on the ground. The key is to use all five senses to take in your surroundings. This is not a time for a photo shoot or Instagram post, though you could capture a picture at the end of your "bath" to spark your memories later.

If you have local nature trails or a park, take a break and go exploring. No soap or towel is needed for this activity as you are bathing your inner being with the refreshing smells, tantalizing sounds, and diverse colors and shapes of nature.

Florence Williams, author of *The Nature Fix: Why Nature Makes Us Happier, Healthier and More Creative*, says that you can "walk into a forest and within five minutes your body and brain start to change. Your heart rate slows. Your facial muscles start to relax. Your hard-working frontal lobes begin to quiet down, and this will boost your productivity and creativity later in the day."

Williams found that current neuroscience studies are giving us the tools to test how things like the smell of trees, quiet green space, and natural views affect the brain. These studies show that as little as fifteen minutes in the woods reduces levels of cortisol, the stress hormone. Increase nature exposure to forty-five minutes, and most people experience improvements in cognitive performance. Even the simple smell of pine trees can boost your immune function.

No forests in your area? That's okay. Finding a place to stand or sit and breathe deeply under a single tree can provide some benefit. You can enhance this limited access with the use of essential oils from the conifer trees mentioned above, plus rosemary. These can be diffused in a room or through a diffusing necklace or bracelet worn on your body. Some studies indicate that adding frankincense to any of these further amplifies the effect.

In conjunction with forest bathing, or even as a simpler starting point, you can consider exploring the practice of grounding that I mentioned in Chapter 14. This practice involves standing or walking barefoot on the ground—in grass, dirt or the sand on the beach. Committed scientists are working to awaken our skeptical world to a forgotten fact: that the Earth beneath our feet contains healing energy, and that connecting ourselves to this energy is remarkably beneficial.

Earthing enables free negative electrons from the Earth's surface to spread over and into your body where they can have antioxidant effects by neutralizing the positively charged free radicals that are so prominent in our bodies. One of many studies demonstrated that earthing reduced inflammation and pain and increased the rate of wound healing.

If your urban environment provides limited options, either look for a small patch of grass or sit in your basement with your bare feet on the concrete floor. Perhaps not as appealing a texture as grass or sand, concrete does allow the electrons to pass from the Earth to your body.

I introduced this concept to one of my clients who suffered from back pain. We talked about the options for her to walk outside in her yard or even sit in a chair with her bare feet on the ground. She lived in a swampy area in south Louisiana where the idea of walking barefoot in her yard did not appeal because of the "creepy crawlies" that abounded. She decided to begin by placing a chair on the concrete slab beneath her raised house where she would spend time sitting in the morning. Within a few days of beginning this practice she noticed that she felt calmer and had less pain.

One of the other benefits of getting out in nature is exposure to sunshine. I think you would agree that a string of cloudy, rain-drenched days can have a depressive effect on your mood. All too often, we spend our days indoors with artificial lighting that does not provide the ultraviolet rays or the brightness of the sun. Combine your earthing with sunshine and you will reap the benefits of the balancing electrons as well as a boost in serotonin and Vitamin D from the sun. Keep your earthing session to fifteen minutes or less (to minimize sunburn risk) and avoid wearing sunglasses or sunscreen to maximize the added benefits of the sunshine.

Those living in more northern climates where winter days are particularly brief may find themselves suffering from Seasonal Affective Disorder, with the appropriate acronym SAD. Their bodies are more sensitive to the lack of sunlight. Making a point to spend an hour outside each day can help, and when this isn't practical, tabletop bright white lights placed nearby can make a big difference.

Electromagnetic exposure from wireless devices, cell phone towers, radios and other modern technology saturates our environment. In our homes and workplaces, we are also subject to recirculated air, chemicals and artificial lighting. Making a point to get outside for forest bathing and grounding breaks give us a way to center our bodies in connection with the Earth and reset our natural electromagnetic fields. The benefits for body, mind and spirit are multiplied

Put into Action

Pause and evaluate what your current situation is. Do you spend much time outside in connection with the Earth? If not, where can you find a suitable outdoor space to sit or walk in the presence of trees and nature? Plan when and where you will explore this valuable connection repeatedly and observe your body's response.

Express Yourself

Have you ever heard of expressive writing? It is defined as personal and emotional writing without regard to punctuation or grammar. Thinking back to days in English class, just this definition sounds freeing. It is more relaxed and unstructured than even a journal or diary, providing a way to essentially "dump" your thoughts and feelings onto a page.

James Pennebaker, professor at University of Texas, got married right out of college in the 1970s. Within just three years, he and his wife were beginning to question their relationship. Insecure and uncertain, Pennebaker began to sink into depression, leaning on drinking and smoking to soothe his doubt.

One morning, with the weight of what he viewed as emotional weakness pressing heavily on him, Pennebaker sat down at his typewriter. After staring at the keys as though in limbo, he put his fingers in place and began pouring out his feelings about his marriage, his parents, his career and even death.

He continued to write in the days that followed and discovered his depression lifting and a fresh clarity in its place. He reconnected with his deep love for his wife and discovered a new direction for his work.

In the four decades that followed, Dr. Pennebaker studied the effect that expressive writing had on people in widely varied situations. His method was to divide them into two groups, one of which would write about emotionally charged events in their lives, while the other group wrote about common things. They would all focus on writing for twenty minutes for three days.

If you have already been in the habit of writing down your thoughts and feelings, this may seem like common sense, but at the time this was revolutionary science. Over and over, the studies clearly demonstrated that the people who wrote about emotional events in their lives experienced less anxiety and depression and reported feeling happier. Following them for months after the writing sessions revealed improved physical symptoms and closer relationships.

The National Institute of Health found a link between depression and early childhood trauma. Strong emotions felt in childhood that are not processed effectively are stored at the cellular level and can cause physical distress later in life. The work of Dr. Pennebaker and others has revealed that expression of those emotions from childhood trauma can work like a pressure valve and release the body from their effect.

Dr. Candace Pert, neuroscientist and author of *Molecules of Emotion: Why You Feel the Way You Feel*, believed that all emotions are healthy, and that they unite the mind and the body. Though we consider some—such as anger, sadness, and fear—to be negative emotions, they are just as valuable to our health as joy and happiness. When we suppress any of our emotions, it creates stress in our body that is reflected in blockages that slow the flow of resources to our cells. Feeling and acknowledging our emotions is honoring ourselves authentically. Releasing them can be vital for health.

Beth, one of the cancer patients I interviewed, shared that as she started treatment, she recognized that she was feeling emotionally drained as well as physically tired. She had heard about the practice of expressive writing and began to write about the treatment process, what was required to coordinate doctors' appointments and recovery time, what she was feeling about it all and why she felt that way. She realized that she was feeling unsupported by her partner as well as the treatment staff, and that she felt gagged so that she couldn't speak up about it. After working through her feelings in writing, she was more relaxed and able to talk with her partner about her needs as well as ask the treatment staff to provide more information about what was planned in coming weeks. This practice of writing about her situation and the feelings it evoked, allowed her to broach her concerns from a level platform rather than the craggy cliff of raw emotion.

I encourage you to explore expressive writing for yourself. Not in an effort to judge your feelings, but simply to bring awareness and acceptance to what may have been bottled up inside you for years. Take a cue from Dr. Pennebaker in how to approach this practice:

1. Set a timer for twenty minutes.
2. Take out a notebook or paper—or open a document on your computer. If writing or typing are not comfortable, you can use a voice recorder and talk it out.
3. When the timer starts, write or talk about your emotional experiences from the past week, month or prior year. Don't worry about punctuation or grammar. Simply go wherever your mind takes you with curiosity and no judgement.
4. Write for an audience of one—yourself—for several days.
5. Then tear the pages out of the notebook and throw them away or close the document without saving it. Those thoughts are now out of you and on the page. They are not intended to be read by anyone else, but simply poured out of your mind and body as you explore them.

You have begun the process of "stepping out" of those experiences to gain perspective. Whether you understand your thoughts or feelings better or not, you have released the pressure and your body can now relax from the stress that the emotional pressure caused.

If you have found this practice beneficial, you can certainly continue. Perhaps this expressive writing will help you process emotions closer to the event in which they were experienced so you reduce the effect that they have on your body. There may be other forms of expression that will allow you to pour out your emotions in various art mediums or dance. This is your expression—*how* you do it is not as important as *doing* it.

Put into Action

Give yourself the gift of three consecutive days of expressive writing as Dr. Pennebaker outlined. On the fourth day, write about the changes you notice in your thoughts and inner being.

Reduce Your Toxin Exposure

CANCER TREATMENT PUTS A GREAT DEAL OF STRESS ON THE body. Compared to life before your diagnosis and the beginning of treatment, there is now far more bombarding your body, as well as your mind and spirit. How are you faring?

Remember when I spoke in the opening chapters about the recluse in the apartment complex, the one that hid from the police patrolling the area? It was a metaphor for the tumor(s) in your body.

Yet there is another reclusive family of which you need to be aware. They come and go in our apartment complex without our realizing, and they can have negative effects if allowed to proliferate. I'm talking about chemicals that permeate our foods (we've already talked about these), our water and air, and our personal hygiene products.

You may be thinking, "Wait a minute, chemicals have been around for decades. What is the problem?" The problem is that the vast majority of these chemicals, which are found in numerous products we use daily, have not been tested for long-term safety. More troubling is the fact that recent testing has shown that a number of them disrupt the function of your hormones, and several have even been identified as carcinogens (cancer causing) but have yet to be taken off the market.

While all but 11 chemicals are allowed in the US, many are not permitted in other countries. The European Union is known for having banned 1300 chemicals, including parabens, phthalates, formaldehyde, triclosan and petroleum distillates.[38, 39] It is a disturbing disparity.

Some of these troublesome chemicals are in our food, but we experience far more exposure from our environment and the products we put on our skin. Did you realize that your skin is a big mouth, absorbing 60% of what is put on it within seconds? I've seen a variety of reports that estimate the average woman being exposed to more than 168 chemicals each day just in her personal hygiene routine. Eeek! And guys, lest you think you are safe because you use fewer products, you are still exposed to an average of eighty-eight chemicals a day.

How can this be permitted? It's all tied up in regulatory red tape. The Food, Drug, and Cosmetic Act was put into law in 1938 (yes, that long ago!) and has not been significantly updated since that time. The Food and Drug Administration (FDA) has been tasked with ensuring that food additives, color additives and pesticides cause "no harm," but they are not authorized to regulate chemicals and contaminants in cosmetics and personal hygiene products. Lest you thought that products wouldn't be on the shelves if they could harm you (as I did when I was a young adult)—that's just not the truth.

I couldn't possibly outline all of the problem children from this recluse family,[40] but I will name a few so that you understand what's hidden behind their hard-to-pronounce names:

Parabens

Parabens—more specifically quadruplets named Methyl-, Ethyl-, Butyl- and Propylparaben—are used as preservatives in cosmetics and personal hygiene products. They are hormone disruptors, meaning that they interfere with proper action of hormones in the body. Through this disrupting activity, they may contribute to sterility in males and early puberty and hormone imbalance in females.

Phthalates

Phthalates are plasticizers and scent chemicals that are found in home products (plastics, carpet, vinyl flooring, air fresheners, and laundry detergent) and personal care products (soaps, shampoos, hair sprays, nail polish, and more). Health effects include kidney and liver damage, birth defects, decreased sperm count, and hormone imbalance. If a product promotes long-lasting scent, put it down and run!

Triclosan

Triclosan is a synthetic antibacterial ingredient that is actually classified as a pesticide by the EPA. It was removed from hand sanitizers but continues to be used in toothpaste, shampoo, deodorants, cosmetics, and other antimicrobial products. Why the FDA won't allow this chemical to be used in antibacterial soaps and gels but considers it fine to use when brushing our teeth is beyond me. Triclosan is classified as a chemical suspected of causing cancer in humans and I do not understand why it continues to be allowed in daily products.

Sodium Lauryl (or Laureth) Sulfate

Sodium Lauryl (or Laureth) Sulfate is a foaming agent used in car washes, engine degreasers and 90% of personal-care products that foam—think shampoo and toothpaste. It's messy stuff that has been attributed to eye damage, depression, diarrhea, skin irritation, and labored breathing.

Polyethylene Glycol

Polyethylene Glycol (PEG are its initials) is used as a thickener, softener and penetration enhancer in skin care, cosmetics, baby wipes, and cleaners. Not only is it contaminated with compounds associated with cancer, but it enhances the penetration of other toxic ingredients included in the products we use.

Ethanolamine

Ethanolamine—triplets Mono-, Di - and Triethanolamine—are foam boosters that cause skin and eye irritation and contact dermatitis. These triplets absorb through the skin and accumulate in organs and the brain. They don't play well there.

THIS IS JUST A SAMPLING OF THE MEMBERS OF THIS RECLUSE chemical family, but I daresay you have an idea of the danger they represent. You can't change the exposure you have already experienced, but you can prevent further exposure now that you know.

Shall we make this a game? Let's go on a scavenger hunt, starting in your bathroom. You might want to have a magnifying glass handy as some products put ingredients in very small print.

Begin scanning the ingredients that are listed on your products. You don't need to be able to pronounce them—thankfully—just spot them. When you see them, set that product off to the side and move to another one. There will be some, like soap and cosmetics for which you no longer have packaging. You can look these up online to check their ingredients or enlist the assistance of a friend or family member to help you with that search. They would benefit from learning what you are discovering too.

At the end of your scavenger hunt, do you find you have very few products that don't have these troubling chemicals? Not unusual at all, since these chemicals are so prolific.

Look at the products you have collected and begin to separate them into ones that you use daily (especially multiple times a day) and less often. If you need to prioritize what products you replace, go for the ones used most often.

Soap is a great place to start. I recommend that you avoid antibacterial soap altogether as the good old-fashioned lye-based soap will do the job quite effectively. Buy a homemade soap that is either unscented or you confirm is not scented with a phthalate-based artificial scent. I provide some resources on my book portal if you need ideas.

Toothpaste is another easy swap. I look for a toothpaste that does not have fluoride, triclosan, or sodium laureth/laurel sulfide in it. You won't find these in the dollar store because cheaper products are made with inexpensive chemicals from this reclusive family, but your health is worth a few more dollars at the checkout.

Related to products that you may not connect with the members of this reclusive family, I also suggest that you explore your home for scented candles and air fresheners. The scent in these is almost always produced with phthalates and you have read the many negative effects they bring. You may be doubtful because you have used these products for quite a long time and not noticed any issues—but are you certain that you are not actually experiencing the ill effects, and is it worth the risk? Diffusing essential oils or burning beeswax candles is a much safer way to shift the scent in a room. In fact, burning beeswax emits negative ions into the air which attracts the positive ions in allergens and pollutants to be burned in the flame or fall to the floor where they are not easily inhaled.

Exploring the incursion of potentially toxic chemicals can feel a bit like opening Pandora's box, yet it is an important first step in ensuring a reduced toxic burden on your body. This, in turn, allows your body to focus more attention on clearing retained toxins rather than dealing with a steady influx of new ones. Each step you take to remove chemicals from the environment and the body in which you live, will make a difference in the way your body functions.

Put into Action

Did you do the scavenger hunt? Think of the value to your body when you identify and eliminate products that are adding harmful chemicals with frequent use. Perhaps it's a project to do with a friend or family member.

Explore Other Forms of Support

IN THE WESTERN CULTURES, WE HAVE LONG LOOKED TO THE medical profession for answers related to our health. While these professionals who devote years to learning about the body are able to assist us, there are other forms of support, some of which have been around for centuries, that are also beneficial for wellness. These would include yoga, meditation and sound baths.

I don't know whether it was the Bible that first introduced to concept of humans being body, mind (or soul) and spirit, but that is where I first heard this foundational truth. Medicine can work on the body, but has recognized its limitations when the soul or spirit of the patient is troubled. A groundbreaking study by the Center for Disease Control and Kaiser Permanente in the mid-1990s revealed the role of childhood emotional trauma in later health challenges and has spurred further exploration.

What doctors and scientists once referred to dismissively as placebo—meaning an outcome based on the patient's belief or perception rather than a causative ingredient—is now being recognized as a valuable aspect of the healing journey that involves both the mind and the body. What you believe about the efficacy of treatment and your body's ability to heal will definitely influence your outcome.

The concept of mind-body medicine and placebo reflects back to the energetic aspect of our bodies, and the way that energy communicates within us. Just like the practice of forest bathing and grounding are recognized to conduct beneficial energy to our bodies, there are other practices that can work with the energy field within and around you.

Yoga

The practice of yoga may be familiar to you, but have you had experience with it? As with exercise, there are many forms of yoga, some calming and others quite active. Some practice yoga for its spiritual principles, while others simply appreciate the many benefits experienced in mind and body. Though I enjoy active exercise, I find my yoga class to be centering and calming with the focus on the breath and listening to my body.

If you are curious about incorporating yoga, I would encourage you to ask your friends or family what classes they like and visit one that interests you. Your cancer treatment may have caused some limitations in movement, so it would be important to speak with the instructor and ensure that they are able to support you with adaptations for some poses. There are also a number of videos online that could give you a taste of the practice. If you are brand new to yoga, I recommend searching for shorter beginner level classes to start.

Imagine my surprise when I learned recently that there is a practice of yoga that is focused on laughter. Created by Dr. Madan Kataria, laughter yoga combines the breathing practices of yoga with the power of laughter, which is good medicine.[41] Just ten-to-fifteen minutes of laughter yoga exercises can reduce stress, make your immune system stronger and keep your mind positive during challenging times.[42] There are many laughter yoga videos available online —check them out and have a good laugh.

Meditation

I've spoken with some patients who felt that meditation made a significant difference in the outcome of their treatment. I find that people have a variety of mental images of meditation. What is yours? Perhaps it's a picture of a monk sitting on the floor staring into space. Or perhaps someone sitting in a tranquil field of wildflowers with an impassive expression on their face. Maybe you are even picturing yourself trying to meditate, grimacing from sitting cross-legged, not to mention being still for ten minutes. I understand, really.

Like so many new explorations, meditation is a practice that starts small and grows with cultivation. In our nonstop culture, stilling the mind does not come naturally. Yet it can develop with practice. Meditation can bring subtle and refreshing nuances to your life—a calmer mind, a new perspective, deeper breathing, and a less frazzled body that is better able to heal. I found it easier to follow a guided meditation when I was starting. There are many apps available: Calm and Headspace are popular, Ten Percent Happier Meditation is good for beginners, and I like Abide for meditation based on Scripture.

If deep breathing is uncomfortable because of mastectomy or removal of lymph nodes, you may find that beginning with meditation will help while your body heals. Once breathing is more comfortable, you could explore yoga more actively.

An unexpected form of meditation that brings mind and body together is the act of coloring. This is a great way to start when you find that just being still is distracting. There are a wide variety of adult coloring books available now—providing a wide range of picture themes—that can aid you in calming body and mind. Whether you use colored pencils, markers or even old-fashioned Crayola crayons because the scent brings back fond memories, sitting down to spend some time coloring is a way to unwind and allow the demands of the world to fall away. No one is pressing you to color within the lines—release the rules that have held you and let yourself go outside the lines if that resonates.

Sound Baths

Some find that incorporating sound in different frequencies deepens the effect of their meditation practice. While forest bathing provides an aspect of sound, there is a practice of sound baths that may speak wordlessly to your body, mind and spirit.[43] A sound bath is an opportunity to break free from daily hubbub to experience deep healing on a cellular level through vibration, which is the essence of sound.

During sound baths, participants settle on a mat with a pillow and blanket and soak up the vibrations from crystal singing bowls, gongs, drums, flutes or other instruments. Each experience varies depending on the instruments and the frequencies used, and how they translate for the individual. Some fall asleep, while others find the music helps them process emotions that may have been buried. It would be ideal for you to experience a sound bath in person near your home. If that is not available, you can look online for a recording. In this case, I would recommend that you use noise cancelling headphones while you are listening to the recording in order to get as close to the immersive experience as possible.

WHETHER YOU USE A MEDITATIVE ACTIVITY, NATURE, SOUND, OR the spoken word as you explore a meditation practice, I appreciate what Bob Sharples shares about meditation. "Don't meditate to fix yourself, to improve yourself, to redeem yourself; rather do it as an act of love, of deep warm friendship to yourself. It offers the possibility of an end to the ceaseless round of trying so hard that wraps so many people's lives in a knot. Instead, there is now meditation as an act of love. How endlessly delightful and encouraging."

So much of your focus in your healing journey may be directed at fixing yourself. Here, you are encouraged to view meditation as simply loving yourself, which may very well be the foundation of healing.

You have the power to listen to your body and choose what you feel would best support you for healing. As you read above, it's not a matter of improved performance, it's a matter of loving your body and supporting it in your journey.

Put into Action

Give yourself the gift of exploring one of these practices as a form of love and friendship with yourself. Once is not enough, though. What will you employ as a practice?

Harness Your Mind
and Body Together

What do you think of when you hear the word *PLACEBO*? In the medical or scientific professions, this word refers to a substance having no pharmacological effect but given merely to satisfy a patient who supposes it to be medicine. It also referred to patients with supposedly malleable minds.

Mind-body medicine is now an emerging area of healthcare in which specialists believe that thoughts and emotions influence healing and well-being. Western medicine usually focuses on treatment of the physical body without considering the impact that emotions, thought and spirit have on the healing process.

Beginning in the 1960s, the scientific literature has grown into a robust collection that clearly demonstrates the power of mind-body techniques to balance the over-activity of the sympathetic nervous system, which is implicated in physical disease. More recently, the literature has been demonstrating beneficial changes in the body's responses affecting hypertension, chronic pain, insomnia, post-traumatic stress disorder (PTSD), and even cancer.

Numerous studies have demonstrated that patients with different forms of cancer who began a mindfulness meditation program reported feeling less stressed and sleeping better. Notably, their immune systems responded to the practice as well, with white blood cells, including the important natural killer cells, rebounding to a normal profile that supported their battle against cancer.

It is also widely recognized that stress—a neurological effect—can cause disease. However, there is a combination of skepticism or cynicism when it is proposed that neurological effects of belief can also promote healing.

As Jo Marchant proposed in her book, *Cure*, "Might the placebo effects, instead of being an illusion that we should puncture, sometimes be of real clinical value? And if it is, can we harness it without exposing patients to potentially risky treatments? Or put another way, can a simple belief—that we are about to get well—have the power to heal?"[44]

Our brains are amazing in their functional capacity and science is regularly discovering that we don't consciously utilize all that is available. Scientific studies have clearly demonstrated that the brain can fill in missing data even where our vision does not capture it, including being able to "see" and react to facial expressions even when there is no visual input.

Collecting data from our senses as we navigate life from birth, our brains continuously anticipate "what we will see, hear or feel next. If parts of an image are obstructed, we still have precise expectation[45] of what the whole object will look like," reports Dr. Lars Muckli of the Institute of Neuroscience and Psychology.

It's clear, then, that our brains are in a near constant state of anticipation. But how does this connect to the placebo effect?

Many practitioners over the years have viewed placebo philosophically as a valuable but annoying effect to overcome. In 1955, it was used to distinguish pharmacological effects from the effects of suggestion. More recently, examining placebo was used to separate out the power of positive thinking. But why seek to eliminate the effect? Why not celebrate that power and put it to use for greater benefit?

Contrary to the assumption that placebo is just people imagining they feel better, placebo effects are genuine, biological effects with a measurable response in the body.

The effect is influenced by the entire therapeutic encounter—highly influenced by the believability of the therapy but even more so by the interaction of the practitioner with the patient. A patient's expectation of positive outcome and their perception of warm care are powerful.

What was your experience with your doctor when you were informed of your cancer diagnosis? Did your doctor simply lay out the facts and answer your questions matter-of-factly, as though you were a number rather than a person? Or did your doctor do so in a manner that helped you see a possible positive outcome and believe that you had an advocate and supporter who would help you recover? Your perceptions in that encounter may have laid the groundwork for placebo to work in your favor. Grasp that and hold on.

If your experience when you learned of your diagnosis was not positive, all is not lost. You can rewrite the story—and even change the people on your team if you do not feel heard or seen as a person—to put the benefits of mind-body medicine[46, 47] to work on your behalf.

What's important to know is that mind-body medicine and your drug-based treatment plan are not mutually exclusive. There is evidence that harnessing the placebo effect can increase the efficacy of a drug or allow consistent effects with a lower or less frequent dose. The good news: you can choose "yes and ...," just as you can choose some of the other tools I have introduced to support your whole being.

One of my clients came to me during a difficult period of her life. Her parents' health was deteriorating, and they needed around-the-clock care. Though my client had the help of care providers, she had to drive several hours every two weeks to check on them, restock groceries and take her parents to medical appointments. There was always a long list of tasks to be accomplished in the two days she was there, and her stress levels were taking a toll. She didn't see another way to meet her parents' needs so we focused on supporting her. She shifted her diet to eliminate foods that worked against her body, boosted some nutrients her body needed, and walked outdoors each morning. When I suggested seeing an acupuncturist, I wasn't sure she would be open to it, but she decided to try it. After just one session, she felt more relaxed and continued to use this therapy regularly.

Even a tool that seems outside your comfort zone may hold the answer for shifting your journey. The key is to invite your mind to be a positive participant in the journey and to educate it on both the possibilities and your belief in your ability to heal.

Put into Action

What will you try? Exploring ways to reduce the effects of stress on your mind and body is vital, and that may involve different forms of support from those shared in Chapter 21 to mindfulness practices. If the situation when you learned of your cancer diagnosis was less than positive, I would suggest that you start with rewriting that story in order to incorporate placebo into your journey.

Break Free of Inner Bonds

RECEIVING A DIAGNOSIS OF CANCER CAN STOP US IN OUR TRACKS. Patricia, one of the ladies I interviewed, said it was like looking at the chart in the eye doctor's office while he changed the lenses. One minute the chart seemed fairly clear and then suddenly it was a blur.

Emotions swirl through shock and disbelief to fear and even anger. The path you had planned has suddenly become strewn with obstacles. Roots, boulders, and overhead branches threaten your steady progress, and you flounder in uncertainty.

Yet with this diagnosis, this unexpected journey, you also have an opportunity. At the end of our conversation, I asked Patricia if there was anything else she wanted to share.

She nodded and paused, then quietly said, "Facing the possibility of death helped me let go of the outer stuff I had collected like a costume for the sake of others, and brought me closer to who I really am."

This is your chance to unzip your carefully curated outer self and step out of that costume to begin to discover the real you.

How you go about this discovery is your choice. While it may feel like you are backed into a corner or being swept downstream in a

strong current, you are empowered with choices all along this path—
what kind of treatment to pursue, the team you that will support you,
the way you will support the whole you along the journey.[48] These
are just a few of the choices you can make. You can choose how, and
even *if*, you peel out of your costume, whether you have help and the
pace at which you do so.

These costumes may have been created by beliefs we have held
on to for years. They are often started in our very early years when
we were learning to navigate our surroundings and stay safe.

Many of us harbor conscious and subconscious memories of past
events. These events may have imprinted a perception or belief that
is still influencing our thoughts and actions today. What I have
discovered in recent years is that many of the beliefs that were
imprinted for me were not actually true. They were a child's
mistaken assumptions from a single event that has held me captive for
decades. And I have yet to meet anyone who doesn't have them incorporated as part of their costume that is keeping themselves hidden
inside.

A significant belief that limited me for decades of my life was
not feeling worth full price. My mother grew up during World War
II and her parents struggled to feed and clothe their large family.
This imprinted stories on my mother who became very frugal. I
remember shopping one day when I was about seven years old and
finding a dress at Hit or Miss (a discounted clothing store) that I just
loved. I showed my mother the dress and begged her to buy it for me.
She checked the price tag and responded that we could make a dress
like it for less than that (discounted) price. Unbeknownst to me, I
decided at that time that I was not worth full price. That story
running in my subconscious drove me to work very hard to save
money and find the best deal on things that I bought. And later, in
my coaching practice, I found it difficult to charge normal prices for
my services.

If this is the first time you've heard this concept, you may be
wondering how you will identify and rewrite those mistaken beliefs

as you peel out of your costume. I can share a few steps that have been helpful for me.

The next time you find yourself dwelling on a circumstance that seemed unfair, or caused you pain, take a moment to become still. Silence and stillness can feel scary if you want to avoid thinking about a situation, yet the only way to break free of that situation's grip on you is to face the emotions that come up and choose to let them go.

Sit quietly in a place without distractions and focus on your breathing. When you visualize that scene in your mind, try to observe it from a different perspective, whether an onlooker or another person that was involved. Acknowledge the emotions you feel, but don't let them take control. Focus on seeing the different perspectives in the scene to explore what was at play.

Take some paper and write down the emotions you are feeling. Pour them out without concern for spelling or grammar. Then take a deep breath or two and look at what you wrote. Ask yourself whether holding on to these emotions is serving a good purpose or actually hindering you.

Full transparency? For me, the vast majority of the time I have done this, I realize that harboring that story and the emotions—anger, sadness, sorrow, rejection, jealousy, etc.—it stirs up are only hurting me. It may be a challenge but be really honest with yourself about why you have held on to the story. Then make the decision to release it, and yourself.

You may find it beneficial to write the story from a different perspective you gained as you observed the scene while sitting quietly. Think about other times in your life when you did something that was the opposite of your original story—something that would disprove what you have believed. Add that into this new story that you are writing. This practice will serve to rewrite the story with the truth that you can now see as an adult. In fact, having this to read repeatedly will help you fix the new story in your subconscious mind to complete the process of breaking free. It may take time to fully release the old story and adopt the reframed story. Awareness is the starting point, and each time you catch yourself thinking or saying something based on the old story, stop and reframe it.

You may want support to help you identify and rewrite those subconscious stories. I have provided some resources for practitioners who specialize in rewriting subconscious beliefs in my book portal that you can explore.

Peeling away the layers of your outer costume is a healing process in itself, involving your emotions and your spirit, which will then—because of mind-body connection—translate to your body. Avoiding the process would keep you zipped up in that costume that doesn't represent who you really are, when the world needs the real you to come forth and shine your light.

Put into Action

You may have felt uncomfortable as you read this chapter and the exercise I suggested. I understand, as I have been there too. Yet I can say from personal experience that committing to the exercise and seeking support in releasing these limiting beliefs and stories, will remove a weight from you that you didn't realize you were carrying. Clear the smudges and dirt that have hindered a clear view of you and past experiences, so that the real you can shine through.

The Greatest of These

In pursuing healing, you would probably agree that it requires more than yourself. You need help in so many different areas. The medical community speaks primarily to the body and what they can influence in your physiology. We've already talked about areas that go beyond this in mind-body medicine and working deeper in your subconscious.

I believe there is also a need to stretch beyond yourself to recognize that you are part of something far bigger than you. We are made for connection—in personal relationships and community. Connection to a higher power will also take you farther than you can go on your own. You are body, soul and spirit, and you are connected (whether you recognize it or not) to spirit. I call that spirit, God, though you may have another term like source or the universe. I believe we were created for relationship with God and until we recognize and pursue that relationship, we will continue to search.

As a believer in God, I consider the Bible to be my roadmap for life. Admittedly, I would like it to be more succinct in instructions for daily living, yet it does provide guidance. Whether you read the Bible yourself of not, you have probably heard the verse from Corinthians

1:13—often called the love chapter—that says, "Faith, hope, and love remain, but the greatest of these is love." Let's explore this a bit, starting with hope.

Have you ever felt that the world's definition of hope seemed rather nebulous? Dictionary.com defines hope as "the feeling that what is wanted can be had or that events will turn out for the best." In a time when emotions can be quite fluid, as during a health crisis, basing hope on feelings doesn't give you a very firm footing. Webster's dictionary defines hope as "a desire accompanied by expectation of or belief in fulfillment." This resonates with me as having a better foundation. Does Webster's definition resonate more with you too?

There's an interesting, though perhaps troubling, story from a study done in the 1950s in which rats were placed individually in large buckets of water to test how long they could tread water. In the first round, the rats lasted just ten to fifteen minutes before sinking to the bottom and drowning. In the second round of the test, the scientific team watched the rats in the buckets and just as the rats gave up, they were plucked out of the water, dried off, and allowed to recover before being put back in the water. How long do you think the rats lasted the next time? Five minutes ... ten ... fifteen? Would you believe forty to sixty *hours*?

What changed for the rats the second time? The introduction of hope. Those that died relatively quickly in the first round gave up mentally rather than physically. But the rats that were rescued in the second round lasted far longer because they had hope of being rescued again. Though disturbing in its methodology, this experiment was a dynamic illustration of the power of hope. The rats had experienced rescue and simply believing it would come again greatly extended their physical stamina.

The Bible defines faith as "the substance of things hoped for, the evidence of things not seen." As we saw with the rats, their faith that rescue would come again was the foundation of their hope. How do we build faith? Like building muscle in our body, building faith requires nourishment and exercise.

You nourish your faith by exploring—talking with others (no doubt, you have been talking to other patients or those who have completed treatment) to collect stories of triumph, or reading the Bible, grasping hold of its promises, and talking with those who are further along in their faith journey than you are. As you talk with others, it is important to be filtering what you hear by keeping what lifts you and releasing the stories that pull you down.

Exercising your faith can include talking to God—expressing your wins, challenges and hopes, and asking for comfort, strength and assistance. Meditating on the verses you have been reading or an encouraging story you heard from another cancer patient or following a guided meditation on a verse/topic that you need to reinforce, is another way to exercise your faith.

Pat, one of the patients I interviewed, was a first-grade teacher when she went through her cancer treatment. She leaned heavily on her faith, praying about her activities and all decisions related to her treatment. She was able to keep going, even continue teaching, and had peace.

Many would encourage you to spend time with God, which may sound odd since the Bible tells us He is always with us. We've all experienced being in a room with someone and not hearing what they say or noticing their actions. Our mind was focused elsewhere. Perhaps you have read of the importance of being "present" with people during an event as a practice of mindfully connecting with them. Likewise, being mindful of God's presence is key to spending time with Him.

How would you act if you were with a friend or family member? You may chat about things that are on your mind, or you may be quite comfortable being together in silence, yet you are still aware of their presence. With some practice, you can build a similar awareness of His presence and it will reinforce both your faith and hope.

The verse I shared initially stated that "greatest of these is love."

Though a noun, love's true power is found when it is viewed as a verb and put into action. The English language is quite limited in vocabulary related to love, but the Greek shows us many words with different inferences.

We are most familiar with *phileo* (fi-LAY-o) love which refers to an affinity for something or someone. This is generally a reciprocal feeling, one that is a response to how someone treats you or the positive energy you receive from them. It is also the form of love that we are using when we see a friend's new coat or hairstyle and joyfully declare that we "love it."

Jesus introduced us to *agape* (uh-GAH-pay) love, which is selfless, sacrificial and unconditional. Agape is not dependent on the response of another but is a choice that looks beyond another's behavior. Can you think of someone in your life from whom you received this love? Someone who looked beyond your actions to see and love who you are. That was an example of agape love and it provides a firm foundation for life. In my experience with clients, it is those who had someone that stood firmly with them in agape love that were able to overcome very difficult circumstances in their lives.

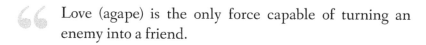
Love (agape) is the only force capable of turning an enemy into a friend.

— Martin Luther King Jr.

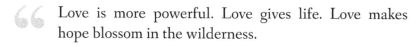
Love is more powerful. Love gives life. Love makes hope blossom in the wilderness.

— Pope Francis

LOVE GIVES LIFE. THAT'S A FORCE I WOULD WANT TO TAP INTO, wouldn't you? What part does love play in your life? Do you focus primarily on *phileo* love, or have you discovered the *agape* love that Jesus introduced? Our human nature would lean toward *phileo*, but the real power is in agape.

Ready for an experiment? Sit quietly and close your eyes. Ask God to show you a person in your life to whom you need to show more love. Then pause and focus. You will see an image in your mind of that person. How can you love them unconditionally? To use a phrase you may have heard before—what would Jesus do to express love to them?

It's possible that you have resistance to loving that person because of an incident with them where you were wounded by their action (or inaction) or perhaps something they said. Sharing life with imperfect humans can be messy. I have yet to meet anyone who hasn't been hurt by someone in their life. This can cause anger or resentment.

Nelson Mandela once said that "resentment is like drinking poison and hoping the other person dies." Who is really hurt by the anger or resentment? Mostly you.

When we have been wounded in some way, it is human nature to hold a grudge. Yet, there are numerous scientific studies that demonstrate the psychological and physiological benefits of forgiveness. These include greater confidence and optimism as well as less stress and pain. Both immune response and cardiovascular health are improved with the act of forgiveness.

In her book *Rewire Your Mind: Discover the Science + Practice of Mindfulness*, Shauna Shapiro writes, "Forgiveness is perhaps the most challenging of all the resources available to us—and the most transformational."

It can be emotionally painful to accept what happened, take radical responsibility for your response to the situation, choose to adopt a new perspective and exercise compassion for the other person in choosing to forgive. It will likely need to be practiced repeatedly each time the situation comes to mind. Over time your emotions will stabilize, and you will be able to observe those emotions as a memory rather than experience them afresh each time you think of the situation. What freedom you will feel as the grip of this unforgiveness loosens and no longer rules your life!

Dr. Frederic Luskin, Director of the Stanford University Forgiveness Project (2003), uses the image of a TV remote control to remind us as we are "surfing" the memories in our mind and come across an area of grievance, to not dwell there. Pause briefly to repeat your forgiveness steps, and then shift your thoughts to things for which you are grateful before you continue surfing. For some, this feels more like a meditation exercise. When you continue to notice the memory, pause, and repeat your choice to have compassion for the person and forgive, the experience loosens its grip on you. There will come a day when you realize you have surfed past an event that used to cause you pain and you can celebrate your growth and healing.

Gratitude carries a power all on its own as we rewrite the stories we carry in our minds. In the process of looking from a new perspective, you may find it helpful to seek small things in the situation for which you are grateful. Focus on the details. For example, if your car broke down, you can be grateful that it wasn't pouring rain and you were able to find help. Expressing gratitude for the clear weather and available help interrupts the negative context of the situation.

One of the ladies that I interviewed viewed her cancer journey as empowering, liberating, refining, hard, and emotional. Do you identify with any of those words? Dawn shared with me that she created ten cancer commandments with the intention that they be guideposts for not allowing her cancer journey to be emotionally debilitating. Her first commandment was "be present and feel all the feels." Rather than stuffing or denying emotions, she gave herself permission to feel them, and then made a point of choosing joy and expressing gratitude every day. Another commandment she wrote was "let my people be who they are," which she said was the hardest one to follow. We all have individuals in our lives who have disappointed us and not provided the support we desired. Dawn recognized that she couldn't hold them in unforgiveness, nor could she allow it to poison her experience, so she needed to release them to be themselves. Do you see that as beneficial for you as well?

As you practice rewriting the stories that have held you back for so long, incorporate gratitude to break the old pattern and identify the positive aspects to include in your new story. Faith, hope, love, forgiveness and gratitude. These are terms you have likely heard all your life, but did you realize they carried such power for transforming your life and the lives of those around you? Give yourself the gift of taking time to ponder and explore new ways to mindfully incorporate these. Not only will this effort contribute to your own wellness, but it can't help but spill out to benefit those around you.

Put into Action

Pull out a piece of paper and reflect on what you have read in this chapter. Write down your thoughts, which of the five—faith, hope, love, forgiveness and gratitude—are in low supply in your life, and how you can begin to bring them in to support your wellness. You may see small steps you can take—write them down and begin to take them.

Reply All

RECALL THE EMAIL I SHARED IN THE INTRODUCTION THAT I received from my friend who was in treatment for breast cancer? She had received a binder with details about her treatment, but all it recommended for nutrition was drinking Ensure or Carnation Instant Breakfast. She reached out to ask my help because she knew there was a better approach and wanted me to join her support team. This book is my response to my friend that I have shared on a broader scale. Instead of just replying to her, I have actually hit "reply all" and you, dear reader, are part of my all.

I hope that in reading these pages you have caught the vision for the power you have to influence your body and the future years of your life. You can control more related to your health and your environment than you may have realized. Your body has amazing powers —far more than our sciences have yet discovered—and using the tools I have shared can support you in your cancer journey and beyond.

At the foundation of that power is the building blocks we provide for our bodies—from the food we consume, to our daily habits and thoughts. All of these provide information for our bodies. Have you noticed as you read those earlier chapters that you may not have been providing quality building materials—good information—for your body to use? You aren't alone. Nor are you stuck where you are. It may not be easy to make changes at first, but each shift you make can make a difference in the function of your body.

You have the power to make different choices to improve the quality of the building materials you are providing to support the non-cancer cells of your body.

Each change you make will shift the way your body functions. Start with the food and beverages you consume, since these are primary sources of building blocks or obstacles for better function. Make different choices with each meal and speak gratitude for the effect those choices will have in your body.

Another key aspect of input for your body is your thoughts, also called your mindset. I shared many sources for identifying and shifting your thoughts, and there are several practitioners linked in the book portal that can further help you. Your body is listening, so be mindful of what you are saying to it in your thoughts and speak kindly with faith, hope, love, forgiveness, and gratitude.

As you embark on this process of supporting your whole being, take time to tune in and notice the changes. Celebrate even the smallest change! That's your body responding. Continue to make different choices and celebrate each change.

Having a buddy can ease the process, whether that buddy is a caregiver, friend or family member. Share this book with them and ask them to help you along the way. It's important that they believe in what you are doing so that they can encourage you when you are tempted to default to old habits.

Dear reader, my greatest desire is that you make choices that empower your body for resilience. Choose love, and gratitude for the lessons you will glean as you walk this journey. When you come out victorious on the other side—I'm holding that belief for you—you will be able to encourage others on their journey.

My friend who launched this project to support you all has now completed her treatment and by the time you are reading this, has had reconstructive surgery. I am delighted to also report that before I finished this book, she married the love of her life and received word from her oncologist that she is cancer free. She is thriving and I seek that for you as well.

Say "yes" to yourself and to making the choices to provide your body the support it needs for life, dear reader! You are precious and loved.

Resources

I have created a book portal as a resource for you. In the portal, you will find videos of many of the chapters from this book for those who are struggling with brain fog, as well as resources that were either mentioned throughout the book or expand on its content. Learn more at www.ThrivingThroughCancerPortal.com or simply use the camera on your phone to snap a photo of this QR code:

Glossary

Adaptogen – a nontoxic plant extract that increases the body's ability to resist the damaging effects of stress and promotes normal function

Angiogenesis – the process of new capillaries forming out of existing blood vessels to supply nutrients to organs and tissues. This is a concern for cancer patients because new capillaries support tumor growth and ability to spread.

Cephalic – of or relating to the head where the senses of sight and smell originate.

Detoxification – the process of separating and removing harmful substances from the body.

Glioblastoma multiforme – the most common and most aggressive form of brain tumor.

Inflammation – an essential part of the body's healing process when injured or infected. External evidence of inflammation would be heat, redness, pain and swelling around a wound. Internal evidence could be fever and pain, but often we aren't aware of ongoing inflammation until disease develops.

Microbiome – a community of microorganisms living in or on the body whose species vary depending on diet, medication, exercise and environmental exposures.

Neurotransmitters – a chemical substance that transmits nerve impulses across a synapse.

Parasympathetic nervous system – is a component of the autonomic nervous system. Together with the sympathetic nervous system, it regulates involuntary and reflexive functions of the human body. The parasympathetic nervous system controls the 'rest and digest' functions, while the sympathetic nervous system control 'fight or flight'.

Semaphore – a system of visual signaling using two flags, one held in each hand

Sleep apnea – a temporary stop in breathing caused by upper airway obstruction during sleep, associated with frequent awakening and often with daytime sleepiness

Endnotes

1. Kumar, Karthik, Allaratha, Shaziya. "Does Sugar Cause Inflammation? Side Effects and More." MedicineNet, September 8, 2022. https://www.medicinenet.com/does_sugar_cause_inflammation/article.htm.
2. Seyfreid, Thomas N. "Cancer As A Mitochondria Metabolic Disease." Frontiers. Frontiers, July 7, 2015. https://www.frontiersin.org/articles/10.3389/fcell.2015.00043/full.
3. Sanchez, Albert, U. D. Register, A. R. Magie, S. Y. Cho, P. J. McMillan, R. E. Willard, P. Y. Yahiku, H. S. Lau, and J. L. Reeser. "Role of Sugars in Human Neutrophilic Phagocytosis." Academic.oup.com. The Journal of Clinical Nutrition, November 1, 1973. https://academic.oup.com/ajcn/article-abstract/26/11/1180/4732762.
4. Shukla, Alpana P., Radu G. Iliescu, Catherine E. Thomas, and Louis J. Aronne. "Food Order Has a Significant Impact on Postprandial Glucose and Insulin Levels." American Diabetes Association. American

Diabetes Association, June 11, 2015. https://
diabetesjournals.org/care/article/38/7/e98/30914/.

5. Takamura, T; Nishino, K; Sakurai, M; Takeshita, Y.
"Consuming Carbohydrates after Meat or Vegetables
Lowers Postprandial Excursions of Glucose and Insulin
in Nondiabetic Subjects." Journal of nutritional science
and vitaminology. U.S. National Library of Medicine.
https://pubmed.ncbi.nlm.nih.gov/30381620/.

6. Yang, Qing. "Gain Weight by 'Going Diet?" Artificial
Sweeteners and the Neurobiology of Sugar Cravings:
Neuroscience 2010." The Yale journal of biology and
medicine. U.S. National Library of Medicine, June 2010.
https://www.ncbi.nlm.nih.gov/pmc/articles/
PMC2892765/.

7. Pearlman, Michelle, Lisa Casey, and Jon Obert. "The
Association between Artificial Sweeteners and Obesity."
Current gastroenterology reports. U.S. National Library
of Medicine. https://pubmed.ncbi.nlm.nih.gov/
29159583/.

8. Walton, R. G., R. Hudak, and R. J. Green-Waite.
"Adverse Reactions to Aspartame: Double-Blind
Challenge in Patients from a Vulnerable Population."
Biological psychiatry. U.S. National Library of Medicine.
https://pubmed.ncbi.nlm.nih.gov/8373935/.

9. Plaza-Diaz, Julio, Belén Pastor-Villaescusa, Ascensión
Rueda-Robles, Francisco Abadia-Molina, and Francisco
Javier Ruiz-Ojeda. "Plausible Biological Interactions of
Low- and Non-Calorie Sweeteners with the Intestinal
Microbiota: An Update of Recent Studies." Nutrients.
U.S. National Library of Medicine. https://pubmed.ncbi.
nlm.nih.gov/32326137/.

10. Soffritti, Morando, Michela Padovani, EvaF Tibaldi,
Laura Falcioni, Fabiana Manservisi, and Fiorella
Belpoggi. "The Carcinogenic Effects of Aspartame: The

Urgent Need for Regulatory Re-EvaluationMorando
Soffritti." American journal of industrial medicine. U.S.
National Library of Medicine. https://pubmed.ncbi.nlm.
nih.gov/24436139/.

11. Daniel, Kaayla, Gregory E Nurse, Sue M., Sunny, Sue
M, CinHus, Carol Holloway, et al. "Why Broth Is
Beautiful: Essential Roles for Proline, Glycine and
Gelatin." The Weston A. Price Foundation, March 15,
2017. https://www.westonaprice.org/health-topics/why-
broth-is-beautiful-essential-roles-for-proline-glycine-and-
gelatin/.

12. Adibi, SA; Wald, A. "Stimulation of Gastric Acid
Secreted by Glycine and Related Oligopeptides in
Humans." The American journal of physiology. U.S.
National Library of Medicine. https://pubmed.ncbi.nlm.
nih.gov/7065145/.

13. Ham, DJ; Murphy, KT; Chee, A; Lynch, GS; Koopman,
R; "Glycine Administration Attenuates Skeletal Muscle
Wasting in a Mouse Model of Cancer Cachexia."
Clinical nutrition (Edinburgh, Scotland). U.S. National
Library of Medicine. https://pubmed.ncbi.nlm.nih.gov/
23835111/.

14. Stehle, P; Kuhn, KS; Muscaritoli, M; Wischmeyer, P.
"Glutamine as Indispensable Nutrient in Oncology:
Experimental and Clinical Evidence." European journal
of nutrition. U.S. National Library of Medicine. https://
pubmed.ncbi.nlm.nih.gov/19936817/.

15. Michalak, Krzysztof Piotr, Agnieszka Maćkowska-
Kędziora, Bogusław Sobolewski, and Piotr Woźniak.
"Key Roles of Glutamine Pathways in Reprogramming
the Cancer Metabolism." Oxidative Medicine and
Cellular Longevity. Hindawi, October 25, 2015. https://
www.hindawi.com/journals/omcl/2015/964321/.

16. Michalak, Krzysztof Piotr, Agnieszka Maćkowska-Kędziora, Bogusław Sobolewski, and Piotr Woźniak. "Key Roles of Glutamine Pathways in Reprogramming the Cancer Metabolism." Oxidative Medicine and Cellular Longevity. Hindawi, October 25, 2015. https://www.hindawi.com/journals/omcl/2015/964321/.

17. Li, Y; Yu, Z; Liu, F; Tan, L; Wu, B; Li, J; "Oral Glutamine Ameliorates Chemotherapy-Induced Changes of Intestinal Permeability and Does Not Interfere with the Antitumor Effect of Chemotherapy in Patients with Breast Cancer: A Prospective Randomized Trial." Tumori. U.S. National Library of Medicine. https://pubmed.ncbi.nlm.nih.gov/17168431/.

18. "Hidden in Plain Sight." SugarScience.UCSF.edu, December 7, 2018. http://sugarscience.ucsf.edu/hidden-in-plain-sight/#.YooS6-jMKo1.

19. "Mushroom Polysaccharide-Assisted Anticarcinogenic ... - Researchgate." https://www.researchgate.net/publication/361566086_Mushroom_Polysaccharide-Assisted_Anticarcinogenic_Mycotherapy_Reviewing_Its_Clinical_Trials.

20. "Mushroom: A New Resource for Anti-Angiogenic Therapeutics - Researchgate." https://www.researchgate.net/publication/339322631_Mushroom_A_New_Resource_for_Anti-Angiogenic_Therapeutics.

21. Kong, Fanming; Tianqi, Chen; Xiaojiang, Li; and Yingjie, Jia. "The Current Application and Future Prospects of Astragalus Polysaccharide Combined with Cancer Immunotherapy: A Review." Frontiers. Frontiers, September 9, 2021. https://www.frontiersin.org/articles/10.3389/fphar.2021.737674/full.

22. Cao, Yihai and Renhai Cao. "Angiogenesis Inhibited by Drinking Tea." Nature News. Nature Publishing Group. https://www.nature.com/articles/18793.

23. "Dietary Prevention of Cancer: Anticancer and ... - Researchgate." https://www.researchgate.net/ publication/233655966_Dietary_Prevention_of_ Cancer_Anticancer_and_Antiangiogenic_Properties_of_ Green_Tea_Polyphenols.

24. Aggarwal, Bharat B.; Shishir Shishodia; Yasunari Takada; Sanjeev Banerjee; Robert A. Newman; Carlos E. Bueso-Ramos; and Janet E. Price. "Curcumin Suppresses the Paclitaxel-Induced Nuclear Factor-ΚB Pathway in Breast Cancer Cells and Inhibits Lung Metastasis of Human Breast Cancer in Nude Mice." American Association for Cancer Research. American Association for Cancer Research, October 20, 2005. https:// aacrjournals.org/clincancerres/article/11/20/7490/ 188552/.

25. A.L. Moseley. "A Systematic Review of Common Conservative Therapies for Arm Lymphoedema Secondary to Breast Cancer Treatment." Annals of Oncology. Elsevier, January 6, 2020. https://www. sciencedirect.com/science/article/pii/ S0923753419378597.

26. Desaulniers, Dr. Veronique. "Easy Ways to Keep Your Lymphatic System Moving." Breast Cancer Conqueror, December 8, 2020. https://breastcancerconqueror.com/ easy-ways-keep-lymphatic-system-moving/.

27. "What Happens When You Sleep: The Science of Sleep." Sleep Foundation, August 29, 2022. https:// www.sleepfoundation.org/how-sleep-works/what-happens-when-you-sleep.

28. "How Does Inadequate Sleep Affect Health?" Eunice Kennedy Shriver National Institute of Child Health and Human Development. U.S. Department of Health and Human Services. https://www.nichd.nih.gov/health/ topics/sleep/conditioninfo/inadequate-sleep.

29. "Blue Light Has a Dark Side." Harvard Health, July 7, 2020. https://www.health.harvard.edu/staying-healthy/blue-light-has-a-dark-side.

30. Fenwick, PB; Ebrahim, IO; Shapiro, CM; Williams, AJ. "Alcohol and Sleep: Effects on Normal Sleep." Alcoholism, clinical and experimental research. U.S. National Library of Medicine. https://pubmed.ncbi.nlm.nih.gov/23347102/.

31. "Why Sitting Has Become the New Smoking." Mayo Clinic. Mayo Foundation for Medical Education and Research, April 5, 2023. https://mcpress.mayoclinic.org/women-health/an-expert-explains-why-sitting-has-become-the-new-smoking/.

32. Menigoz, W; Latz, TT; Ely, RA; Kamei, C; Melvin, G; Sinatra, D; "Integrative and Lifestyle Medicine Strategies Should Include Earthing (Grounding): Review of Research Evidence and Clinical Observations." Explore (New York, N.Y.). U.S. National Library of Medicine. https://pubmed.ncbi.nlm.nih.gov/31831261/.

33. Chevalier, G; Patel, S; Weiss, L; Chopra, D; Mills, PJ. "The Effects of Grounding (Earthing) on Bodyworkers' Pain and Overall Quality of Life: A Randomized Controlled Trial." Explore (New York, N.Y.). U.S. National Library of Medicine. https://pubmed.ncbi.nlm.nih.gov/30448083/.

34. Chevalier, Gaétan; Stephen T Sinatra; James L Oschman; Karol Sokal; and Pawel Sokal. "Earthing: Health Implications of Reconnecting the Human Body to the Earth's Surface Electrons." Journal of environmental and public health. U.S. National Library of Medicine, 2012. https://www.ncbi.nlm.nih.gov/pmc/articles/PMC3265077/.

35. "Castor Oil - Dr. Philip Princetta." https://drprincetta.com/wp-content/uploads/2016/01/Castor-Oil.pdf.

36. "150 Inspiring Quotes on Beating Cancer from Super Survivors - Parade." https://parade.com/1140135/kaitlin-vogel/cancer-quotes/.

37. "Exploring the Nature Pyramid - National Parks Board." My Book.

38. "US Cosmetics Are Full of Chemicals Banned by Europe – Why?" The Guardian. Guardian News and Media, May 22, 2019. https://www.theguardian.com/us-news/2019/may/22/chemicals-in-cosmetics-us-restricted-eu.

39. Campos, Paulina. "9 Beauty Ingredients That Are Banned in Europe (but Legal in the U.S.)." Byrdie. Byrdie, January 28, 2022. https://www.byrdie.com/banned-ingredients-europe.

40. "Chemicals Archive." Safe Cosmetics. https://www.safecosmetics.org/chemicals/.

41. Pruessner, JC; Meier, M; Wirz, L; Dickinson, P. "Laughter Yoga Reduces the Cortisol Response to Acute Stress in Healthy Individuals." Stress (Amsterdam, Netherlands). U.S. National Library of Medicine. https://pubmed.ncbi.nlm.nih.gov/32393092/.

42. Dolgoff-Kaspar R; Baldwin, A; Johnson, MS; Edling, N; Sethi, GK. "Effect of Laughter Yoga on Mood and Heart Rate Variability in Patients Awaiting Organ Transplantation: A Pilot Study." Alternative therapies in health and medicine. U.S. National Library of Medicine. https://pubmed.ncbi.nlm.nih.gov/22894892/.

43. Goldsby, Tamara L, Michael E Goldsby, Mary McWalters, and Paul J Mills. "Effects of Singing Bowl Sound Meditation on Mood, Tension, and Well-Being: An Observational Study." Journal of evidence-based complementary & alternative medicine. U.S. National Library of Medicine, July 2017. https://www.ncbi.nlm.nih.gov/pmc/articles/PMC5871151/.

44. Marchant, Jo. Cure: A Journey into the Scient of Mind Over Body. New York: Broadway Books, 2016, pg 9.

45. "Discovery Shows How Brain 'Fills in Blanks' to Help Us See." ScienceDaily. ScienceDaily, June 2, 2000. https://www.sciencedaily.com/releases/2000/06/000601164617.htm.

46. "Mind over Matter: The Power of Placebo." Psychology Today. Sussex Publishers. https://www.psychologytoday.com/us/blog/surprise/202201/mind-over-matter-the-power-placebo.

47. "The Power of the Placebo Effect." Harvard Health, December 13, 2021. https://www.health.harvard.edu/mental-health/the-power-of-the-placebo-effect.

48. "Quality of Life of Cancer Patients during ... - Wiley Online Library." https://onlinelibrary.wiley.com/doi/full/10.1002/pon.5434.

About the Author

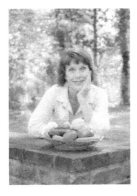

*Photo credit: Still
Reflections Photography*

Kelly Lutman has been fascinated by the power of food ever since she helped resolve her son's ADHD simply by changing his diet. A health coach certified in Applied Functional Medicine, Kelly firmly believes that symptoms are the body's cries for help, and that the body can heal when provided the building blocks it needs. She meets each client where they are, helps them understand what is happening in their body, and guides them in identifying the changes that will help them experience the vitality they were missing. She lives in Slidell, Louisiana, with the love of her life and their family.

Kelly has created a book portal with helpful information to support the contents of this book. Visit www.ThrivingThrough-CancerPortal.com to learn more.

 facebook.com/PursueWellnessForYou

 linkedin.com/in/kellylutman

 instagram.com/kelly_lutman

About the Publisher

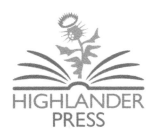

Highlander Press, founded in 2019, is a mid-sized publishing company committed to diversity and sharing big ideas thereby changing the world through words.

Highlander Press guides authors from where they are in the writing-editing-publishing process to where they have an impactful book of which they are proud, making a long-time dream come true. Having authored a book improves your confidence, helps create clarity, and ensures that you claim your expertise.

What makes Highlander Press unique is that their business model focuses on building strong collaborative relationships with other women-owned businesses, which specialize in some aspect of the publishing industry, such as graphic design, book marketing, book launching, copyrights, and publicity. The mantra "a rising tide lifts all boats" is one they embrace.

f facebook.com/highlanderpress
⊙ instagram.com/highlanderpress
in linkedin.com/highlanderpress
⑂ pinterest.com/highlanderpress